ALONE IN MY UNIVERSE:

Struggling with an Orphan Disease in an Unsympathetic World

WAYNE BROWN

iUniverse, Inc.
Bloomington

Alone in My Universe
Struggling with an Orphan Disease in an Unsympathetic World

iUniverse books may be ordered through booksellers or by contacting:

iUniverse
1663 Liberty Drive
Bloomington, IN 47403
www.iuniverse.com
1-800-Authors (1-800-288-4677)

ISBN: 978-1-4502-9592-5 (pbk)
ISBN: 978-1-4502-9593-2 (clth)
ISBN: 978-1-4502-9594-9 (ebk)

Library of Congress Control Number: 2011903805

Printed in the United States of America

iUniverse rev. date: 3/18/11

This book is dedicated to all people who have faced down a disease and all of its complications, having done everything in their power to emerge victorious and to win back their own lives.

It is also dedicated to the people we count on to pull us through our struggles: our families, our friends, our doctors and nurses, and the countless others who help to make our lives better, simply by being part of us. Thank you!

Book Chapters

Foreword

Laurence Katznelson, MD
Stanford University

When faced with a chronic disease such as Acromegaly, a person and his/her family come face to face with a daunting situation. The person (now a patient) must find a way to come to grips with a chronic disease that will encompass an important and large portion of his/her life. This is a very difficult process, and one of the main ways to accomplish this is to obtain information. Information is key, as, once armed with such information, people are in a better position to grasp the implications of this new disease and to help make appropriate decisions. Knowledge of the disease is an important coping method. In my experience, knowledge may be relatively easy to gain if the disease is common, as there are any number of available books, talk shows, internet sites, and health care providers that can provide access to such information. Attaining the critical knowledge is less possible in the presence of an uncommon disease, such as Acromegaly, where such information is less easy to come by. The title of this book, *Alone in My Universe*, says it all: the process of understanding and fighting a chronic disease, particularly one as uncommon as Acromegaly, leaves one with the sense of isolation, with an onslaught of questions on how to fight the battle.

This book serves as a primer for understanding Acromegaly from the viewpoint of patients, with descriptions of coping based on experiences from multiple people. When I was asked to write a foreword for this book, I thought long about how I could best contribute. As an endocrinologist with a specialty in pituitary disorders, I have witnessed many people go through the process of disease diagnosis and therapy, and have seen a spectrum of reactions and coping skills. So, it made sense that where I can contribute the most in this context is through a description of Acromegaly. This way, when someone reads this book, he/she can have a better understanding of the decisions that were made and the outcomes that were achieved.

So, what is Acromegaly? Acromegaly is a chronic, debilitating disease characterized by excessive production of a hormone called growth hormone (GH) by the pituitary gland. The pituitary gland sits in the base of the skull under the brain, in a boney pouch called the sella tercica. The pituitary gland is connected to the base of the brain, at the hypothalamus, by a "stalk," which is filled with blood vessels and nerves that bring important chemicals to the pituitary gland. The pituitary gland is called the master gland, as it produces many of the hormones that control important processes in the body. For instance, the pituitary gland controls production of thyroid hormone (energy and metabolism), LH and FSH (the reproductive, gonadotropin hormones responsible for fertility and sexual function, including estrogen in women, testosterone in men), prolactin (allows for nursing), adrenocorticopin (ACTH, controls production of cortisol, a steroid critical for metabolism and maintenance of blood pressure), antidiuretic hormone (ADH, controls fluid and electrolyte levels), and, lastly, GH. GH is produced in bursts (pulses) through the day, largely at night, and causes the liver to make insulin-like growth factor (IGF-I). IGF-1 serves as a marker for how much GH is present and is also responsible for many of the effects of GH on the body.

In most patients with Acromegaly, there is a benign (non-cancerous) growth (called a tumor or adenoma) of the pituitary gland that produces excessive amounts of GH. High levels of GH lead to elevated levels of IGF-1. Therefore, a diagnosis of Acromegaly is made by measurement of a blood level of IGF-1, and an elevated IGF-1 level helps clinch this diagnosis. GH can be measured as well in the blood, but the standard way of doing this is by measuring blood GH levels following an oral glucose tolerance test. In this test, the person swallows a sugar (glucose) solution, and GH levels are measured over about 2 hours through an intravenous line. If the GH falls below 1.0, then this is considered normal. A GH value above 2 is considered elevated, suggestive of Acromegaly. However, none of these tests are perfect, and even someone with Acromegaly may have a low GH level. Therefore, the diagnosis is sometimes unclear, and referral to an experienced endocrinologist may be the appropriate course. Following confirmation blood testing and a diagnosis of Acromegaly, an MRI scan is performed to look for a pituitary tumor. By the time Acromegaly is diagnosed, these pituitary tumors are often more than 1 cm in length, which is defined as a macroadenoma. If large, the tumor may be pressing on the eye nerves (the optic chiasm above), which may lead to loss of peripheral vision. Many people do not know if they have lost such vision, and they need to see an ophthalmologist for peripheral vision testing. If large enough, the tumor may press on the adjacent, normal pituitary gland, resulting in reduced pituitary hormone production. This means that the pituitary gland is unable to produce one or more of the hormones described above, resulting in hypopituitarism (meaning low pituitary function). If the thyroid hormone is low, the person may need to take a thyroid pill. If the cortisol is low, the patient may need to take a prednisone or hydrocortisone pill. If the female estrogen level is low (such as is seen with loss of menstrual cycles), then estrogen therapy may be necessary. If the male hormone testosterone is low, then testosterone therapy may be necessary. Therefore, pituitary function testing is a routine part of the evaluation.

Because the body changes, including thickened facial bones and enlarged hands and feet, occur very slowly, the diagnosis may be delayed for up to ten years. People usually do not notice the gradual changes. It may be that the diagnosis is considered when someone sees a new doctor, or a long-lost relative or friend, who notices the changes. For example, in the chapter "Managing Disease Symptoms," a woman was introduced to her disease when she saw an old friend (now a physician) at a sorority reunion, and the physician noticed her facial changes. The poignancy of this delay in diagnosis is described so well in this book—from the chapter "Pre-diagnosis and Frustration," where the woman had, in retrospect, many of the changes associated with Acromegaly, but it wasn't until she lost vision that the diagnosis of pituitary adenoma was entertained by an endocrinologist, to the man in "Life around Surgery" who, despite many of the classic findings, endured recurrent and painful spinal disc disease and carpal tunnel syndrome before the diagnosis was considered. This is the usual situation: because it is a rare disease, physicians often spend a career without ever seeing a case and, hence, are not often equipped to make the diagnosis in a timely fashion.

Because of this delay, there are many years for the effects of high levels of GH to affect the body. Patients often describe pain, such as headaches or joint pains. Headaches are a common problem with Acromegaly, and they may be the reason that patients initially seek attention. The joint pains, due to destructive arthritis, may be very limiting and, despite appropriate therapy to treat the Acromegaly, may persist and be a long-term problem. Another medical consequence is sleep apnea syndrome, characterized by snoring and morning headaches and fatigue due to excess swelling of the back of the throat. In addition, Acromegaly is associated with hypertension, type 2 diabetes mellitus, and atherosclerosis, which may all contribute to heart disease. The heart may be thickened due to GH exposure, and the heart may not be able to pump adequately. Patients may notice that they tire easily with exertion, and this may be a sign of underlying heart problems that need to be evaluated and addressed. These associated medical problems may be present in isolation or as a group and may therefore be quite debilitating. It is critical to understand that appropriate therapy may lead to marked improvement in these consequences. For example, diabetes and hypertension may improve and headaches usually resolve with lowering of GH and IGF-1. Sleep apnea syndrome may improve as well, but patients often have residual sleep apnea syndrome despite therapy, so a sleep study with appropriate therapy may be necessary. Another consideration, which is not trivial, is the psychological effect of having distorted features. Patients often describe self-image issues, which may be bothersome and lead to depression. These issues need to be considered as well in the approach to a patient.

Another important medical problem in Acromegaly is the concern for an increased risk of cancer. Colon polyps are often found in patients, and these may be premalignant. There has been a suggestion that the risk of colon cancer is higher in patients with Acromegaly, though this has not been clearly proven. Nevertheless, a screening colonoscopy is recommended to detect and remove polyps, and to search for possible cancer. Another significant concern is the risk of early death, primarily due to heart disease. There have been a number of studies that have now shown that appropriate treatment, with achievement of normal GH and IGF-1 levels, can reverse this risk. Because therapy can lead to dramatic improvement in these medical consequences, appropriate diagnosis and therapy are paramount!

The therapy is tailored to meet the following goals: 1) to normalize the GH and IGF-1 levels, 2) to prevent tumor compression of the local brain structures, and 3) to improve the medical consequences of the disease (described above). Surgery, with an experienced surgeon, is considered the primary therapy and is the only therapy that can lead to rapid and long-lasting normal GH and IGF-1 levels. Surgery is mandated if the tumor is pressing on important structures, such as the eye nerves (optic chiasm), and surgery can result in rapid improvement in vision. The success of surgery is based on the size and position of the tumor. For example, if the tumor is large (macroadenoma) and extends beyond the sella turcica into an area called the cavernous sinus (on the side of the pituitary gland), then the tumor cannot be cured by surgery as this is not an accessible area for a surgeon. If this is the case, then surgery can reduce the size of the tumor, but we know going into the surgery that there will be tumor left, despite the best efforts. As far as the patient is concerned, surgery is an overwhelming consideration, and the experience from the patient's viewpoint is encapsulated nicely in the chapter "Transsphenoidal Surgery, CSF Leak: My Story," where the anticipation and daily postoperative course are charted in a way that adds a human face to the recipient of this procedure. This is a chapter that should definitely be read by physicians.

Medical therapy is usually considered as secondary therapy following failed surgery (although it can be considered as the initial therapy instead of surgery in certain circumstances). The major medical therapy available is that of somatostatin analogs. There are two such medications, octreotide long acting release (Sandostatin LAR®) and lanreotide depot (Somatuline autogel®), which are effective in lowering the GH levels. These medications are very similar in their benefits and risks (including gallstones and gastrointestinal upset, mainly) and are given as monthly injections in the buttock. There are some differences in how they are administered, which may influence availability for patients. Somatostatin analogs are well tolerated overall. In patients with a persistently elevated GH and IGF-1 despite somatostatin analogs, or who do not tolerate these medications, the next drug to consider is pegvisomant (Somavert®), which is a human GH molecule that has been changed and, when given as a subcutaneous injection, blocks all of the GH in the body. Pegvisomant is highly effective, in almost all patients, in lowering IGF-1 to normal. Pegvisomant is well tolerated, though liver tests can become abnormal and there have been rare instances of growing tumor: therefore, both blood liver tests and brain MRI scans need to be followed. Lastly, there are dopamine agonist drugs, including cabergoline (Dostinex®) and bromocriptine (Parlodel®), which are oral and less expensive than the other medications. Though useful, they normalize the IGF-1 values in a minority of people; so, use is limited. Given these medical options, the majority of patients should have a highly successful medical course, and it should be possible to achieve normal GH and IGF-1 levels in most patients.

Lastly, radiation therapy has a role, but largely a secondary one, for treatment of persistent disease despite surgery and/or for treatment of disease that is poorly responsive to medical therapy. There are several types of radiation therapy, including conventional, fractionated radiation therapy where small doses of radiation are given daily for up to 5-6 weeks. This is useful in larger tumors, as well as in centers that do not have access to another technique called radiosurgery (includes gamma knife, proton beam, and cyberknife). Radiosurgery is administered in a single or a few doses, so this may be more convenient for patients. All types of radiotherapy appear to be similarly effective at lowering GH and IGF-1. It needs to be understood that, for all of these techniques, it may take years for the GH and IGF-1 levels to normalize, and a side effect is hypopituitarism. Therefore, normal pituitary function needs to be monitored and hormone replacement should be given if the levels are low.

In summary, Acromegaly is a chronic disease that affects many body systems. With appropriate therapy, many of the signs and symptoms of this disease, as well as medical consequences, can be improved. This often requires a team approach, as there are many medical subspecialities involved in the care. From the patient side, an understanding of these medical issues is so very important for appropriate decision making. As can be seen above, there are a number of decision points in the process, and knowledge of the pros and cons of each treatment is critical for adequate patient input in making these decisions.

Alone in My Universe: Struggling with an Orphan Disease in an Unsympathetic World

I still cannot believe how much a life can change in a very short time. It was a cold and snowy November day in 2004 when my doctor informed me that I was not a hypochondriac. The symptoms I had been complaining about for almost a decade were actually real. That sheer relief I felt when diagnosed was quickly shattered when the word *tumor* rang through my head. Tears of joy were abruptly replaced with abject fear and millions of questions about a disease that, not only had I never heard of, I couldn't even remember the name to try to learn about it!

If you are reading this book, you are most likely somehow involved with Acromegaly. You may be a health care provider, the loved one of a patient, or an Acromegaly patient yourself. Whatever your connection to this disease, we welcome you to come and learn about Acromegaly from the patient's perspective. The intention of this book is for you to find love, support, and encouragement inside of these pages. It was not written to be academic; it is all about mutual support. When we discuss medical issues or procedures in the book, understand that they are being retold from what we have experienced, combined with what our medical professionals have told us. If you read anything in here that is of medical interest to you, please make sure that you discuss it with your trusted medical professional first. None of the writers in this book are Medical Doctors, so please keep that in mind; all stories and experiences are purely anecdotal.

When I was talking with the writers about ideas for this project, I told them that their goal was to write their chapters as if they were telling their story to a newly diagnosed patient who was unsure of his/her future. Write it as if the person reading your chapter was just diagnosed and might be sitting in a waiting room or sitting and waiting for test results to come back.

This book is a collaborative effort from people who have been touched by Acromegaly, none of whom are professional writers. Most of us are patients working to manage a disease that most of us had never heard of before diagnosis. The only contributors involved with this project who are not patients are a professional psychologist, a professional advisor to medical corporations, and a personal friend. The psychologist is working to offer suggestions for disease management as a patient and as a loved one. The friend is writing about dealing with Acromegaly as an outsider who cares about the patient.

The patients who have written full chapters have all chosen a theme to focus on, and they were each guided to tell their own life story as it relates to Acromegaly and its effects, while still focusing on the theme of their chapter. So while one writer will tell their story focusing on their experiences with work issues, another person will tell their personal story focusing on managing negative energy, and others will focus on managing family issues. The Table of Contents will offer you a guide as to what each writer is focusing on. If you choose to read chapters in non-sequential order, the book will still make sense, since each chapter was written individually; please just make sure that you take the time to read each chapter. All of us put a great deal of mental and emotional work into sharing our lives with you, and I believe that this energy comes through loud and clear. If you are a patient, you will probably say “me-too” more than once, and if you are a friend or family member, there will probably be times where you say “no wonder.” You will notice that the chapters are not numbered. This is intentional. Because the chapters do not need to be read sequentially to make sense, numbering the chapters did not seem necessary. Chapter One is just as important as Chapter Seven, and Chapter Four adds just as much to the overall picture as Chapter Twelve. Please do not let this detract from your enjoyment of the book, but let it enhance the idea that all of the stories are equally important to getting the full snapshot of life with a rare disease.

I believe it is that similarity of struggle that binds us all. Whether you are a patient or a loved one of a patient, there is a great deal that can be learned from other people's experiences. While our paths to diagnosis may differ, there is a definite thread of similarity within all Acromegaly patients, and I think it is that similarity that will offer you comfort. While the patient may feel that they are suffering alone, there are many people in our universe who also have to manage the disease from their own perspectives.

To get the perspective of dealing with Acromegaly from the non-patient perspective, I asked some experts to contribute to the dialogue. We are honored to have a lawyer discussing rights in the workplace, a Social Worker sharing how to talk with children about your disease, a medical marketing expert on his experiences dealing with rare diseases, and a psychologist to discuss managing the emotional side of Acromegaly. I also asked a close friend of mine to share his experiences on what it is like to deal with the disease as a friend.

There are two chapters that were designed to draw in even more voices. These stories are shared from individual members of our Facebook group and AcromegalyCommunity.com. One chapter focuses on their individual experiences with the medical community, and the other addresses how parents talked with their children about their disease.

I hope that the diversity of voices in our book will provide knowledge and support for patients and their loved ones. While we are cooperatively raising the awareness of Acromegaly, it is still a very low-profile disease, and I think that is part of our struggle. Up until recently with use of the internet, there were no support networks for people dealing with Acromegaly, and a patient could spend their entire life never communicating with a fellow patient. Thankfully technology has shrunk the globe enough that acromegalics can have friends who are fellow patients.

It is my true hope that you enjoy this book and find ideas and support for managing your disease and mutual support between patients and their loved ones. All people touched by the disease are welcome to join the dialogue at www.AcromegalyCommunity.com. Log on and make friends who understand what you are dealing with.

So why is it called *Alone in My Universe* if there are so many people involved in this project? We have all traveled a very similar path. I think you will discover as you read this book that many of us start down the path of Acromegaly feeling quite lonely. I often remind our members that we are all a family. While we all may have our own natural families, there is a part of us that they can never understand. And up until recently, most of us have never met other patients. When we would try to describe what we were going through, the most we could hope for was a little bit of sympathy. Empathy was impossible since our symptoms are so foreign to most people. We are surrounded by people who love and care for us, yet we still feel completely alone in our universe. As I was working on writing this part of the book, I was emailed a story from a member and a friend. She had shared a piece that I had written on loneliness with a friend of hers. He was so moved that he wrote back to me through my friend with a story of how he described his loneliness of the disease. "I felt like I was with others in a stream. We were crossing the stream. All the others had crossed and were at the opposite bank, but I was slow and struggling in the middle. They cheered me on. *Try harder, you can do this*, they called out. No matter how I struggled, I couldn't move forward, and the water level kept rising. I felt like I would drown…all by myself. The others just watched from the bank, not understanding why I couldn't cross the stream faster and easier." I hope that you find this book helpful. Let it be one of your emotional life rafts to help you sail across the uneasy waters of loneliness.

Thank You

Where to start… Writing my first book required the support of more people than I ever would have imagined. While this project has consumed more than two years of my life, it has been an absolute labor of love, and now that the book has been completed, I am so happy and proud of what all of our writers have accomplished in building *Alone in My Universe.*

The first thanks must obviously go out to the wonderful writers who contributed to this book. When I first went searching for people willing to share their stories, I never would have expected the level of talent and dedication that I found. Moreover, I got to enjoy absolutely fascinating stories of struggle and triumph that really helped me to appreciate my own life and my own struggles and triumphs. I pushed you to share your lives in our pages, in hopes that we could help others battling their own loneliness and isolation. I can say with great confidence that you gave it your everything, and our readers will benefit from your generosity of spirit. Thank you for indulging my endless questions and comments. "Explain," "Why?" and "This is great, but can you add a little more?" were just a few of the regular notes the writers would get back. Sometimes we gave each other static, but the final product shines through the pain. I would like to single out one writer for additional thanks though: Tyson Koerper. He has been volunteering his amazing artistic skills to Acromegaly Community since the very beginning, and when I called on him to turn my somewhat disjointed ideas into a stunning book cover, he listened to everything I said and ran with it. I think you will agree that this book looks beautiful. And I think that you can safely say that in this case, you can indeed judge a book by its cover!

In addition to our official writers, we also have our collaborators. While working on the book, I thought that with some subjects, multiple perspectives were needed, so I asked our members to share their own stories. The two collaboration chapters were all segments submitted from our members in a less formalized structure. All they had to work with were the specific questions of "How did you talk with your children about the disease?" and "How do you personally manage your disease and its side effects?" Their stories offer a wide-ranging glimpse into the daily management of Acromegaly.

I would like to thank two specialists for their generosity of knowledge in helping to round out the book with their brilliant excerpts. Kathy Kurtz, MSW, was kind enough to share knowledge on how to talk to your children about your diagnosis, and Lindy Korn, Esq., contributed an article she wrote on Genetic Discrimination in the workplace. Both were generous in donation of their knowledge and experience for patients in need of both.

I must also thank the great people that helped me get this book ready for publication. As you read the chapters, you will see some very sensitive issues are discussed. I wanted to make sure that all issues were being handled honestly and fairly, since my honesty should not cause anybody else unnecessary discomfort or pain. Thank you to Kathy Kurtz for reading when I had concerns. Your feedback was always helpful and informative. Thanks also to Wendy Sadkin, the only family member who got any previews of the book. You only got to read a small part, with sworn confidentiality! You reassured me that this very delicate part of our family history was handled with the appropriate tact and diplomacy, while maintaining complete honesty about the events that took place. And you kept it all secret, which I really appreciate.

As the book was winding down and we were looking to market it, I was in a totally new area and reached out for help from Gloria Nobleza Wise. She was wonderful in her desire to help when I had questions. And when she didn't have the answer, she knew who did. One of the people she directed me to was Kathryn Radeff. Thank you, Kathryn, for your knowledge and experience. You helped me focus the book so it should appeal to a large audience, without losing the message to our intended audience. And I do think that we successfully accomplished that.

As we faced publishing deadlines, I threw a mountain of work at my friend, and editor, Michelle Smith. She handled it with the poise and aplomb that I have come to expect and deeply respect. Above all, I told her to please make sure to keep the speakers' voices intact, and she did a marvelous job of making sure all stories were understandable and interesting to all readers. Most importantly to me, every time I threw another item at her, or changed a deadline, she smiled and accepted it in stride. I could not have asked for a better person to handle my biggest project.

And when it comes to support, I must give unending thanks to my family and friends. Not only have they watched me toil away at this book for years, they have had to listen to my unending conversations about the book. My sister, Nicole Brown Parrish, and her husband, Greg Parrish, have been amazing in their support, encouragement, and ideas over the years. As to support from friends, Beth Seilberger is the friend who provides good ideas, offers great feedback on writing, and keeps me humble when I need that too. Ray Graf, who is in the book as a writer, has also been one of my most staunch supporters both for the book and for charitable events. Everyone should be lucky enough to have a friend like him in their lives

Last, but certainly not least, I would like to thank you, the reader. You have taken the time to share our lives with us. I hope that you come out with a deeper, more meaningful understanding of the human spirit and its ability to triumph against incredible struggles. That is, after all, what this book is all about. Man vs. Disease. And without exception, every one of these writers has learned to live a normal, functional life in spite of Acromegaly—making us all victorious in our battles. I look forward to the day when you call me and tell me your story of your victory.

Pre-diagnosis and Frustration

Danielle Roberts

We learn geology the morning after the earthquake.
—Ralph Waldo Emerson, *The Conduct of Life*

I must confess that I am not tremendously familiar with the works of Ralph Waldo Emerson, but as I was looking for an appropriate opening for this chapter, I found the above quote and thought it be quite fitting of my journey with Acromegaly. Before Acromegaly, the word *pituitary* just sounded silly to me. It reminded me of what a cartoon character might say while spitting something out due to a foul taste. I had no idea what it was, where it was, or what it did, but I can certainly tell you a thing or two about it now. You tend to learn these things very quickly when a doctor in a crisp white coat says he needs to cut into your head to reach your pituitary.

My name is Danielle, and I'm thirty-two years old. I was diagnosed with Acromegaly in 2002. I still remember the day I received my diagnosis as clearly as if it were yesterday, and it's hard for me to believe that I've been aware of my disease for eight years now. Nearly every acromegalic I know travels a lengthy path toward diagnosis, though most of us only recognize it in hindsight. It is my hope to give the best picture possible of what my path was like, and I believe it's important to share a little bit about my background in order to do that.

When you have any kind of difficult medical condition, your support system is your lifeline, and everybody's support system is a little different. No matter what yours is, you definitely need to have one. At this point in my life, I'm a single adult with no children—though I do have a very spoiled Schnauzer. My lifeline through this journey has been my parents, grandparents, siblings, and close friends. Generally speaking, for one reason or another, I haven't spent too much time focusing on other relationships. I move quite a bit because I enjoy experiencing new places, and romantic relationships have come and gone but have never really gotten too serious for me. Occasionally, when I do start thinking about a romantic relationship with someone new, I always have to address certain questions. When should I tell him about the Acromegaly? Or, what if things get really serious and he wants kids down the road? Honestly, they're not really questions I always know how to deal with. For the most part, though, I try to live one day at a time and not to think about things I can't control in the present. I'm just grateful for the wonderful friends and family in my life who have been there for me in more ways than I can count.

Now that I've given a brief synopsis of my support structure, I should probably move on and tell you a little about how I handle more practical daily things. Everybody has to make a living, and I'm certainly no exception to that rule. Throughout my adventures as an adult, I have always supported myself in administrative roles while dabbling in college as I could afford the time and money to take classes. It's not the traditional way to go about things, but I've never been much of a traditionalist, so it works for me. Additionally, thanks to my Acromegaly, I have to make sure that I always have full-time work to ensure I can maintain health coverage. I hope that one day, healthcare in the United States will actually be affordable and accessible without having to depend on employers for it; but for now, I do the best I can working with the system we have.

I'd like to go back a little further now so I can share some of the frustrations I experienced on the long path toward diagnosis. If you've also been recently diagnosed, I'm sure you'll be spending quite a bit of time looking back on memories of certain situations and just knowing that something wasn't quite right in your body. There are so many signs and symptoms that you can look back and see in hindsight—but you never would have caught them "back then."

Acromegaly is a very slow and sneaky disease. It's hard enough to diagnose on its own disease, but if you are already dealing with other medical issues, it is common to blame the Acromegaly symptoms on the existing conditions. I have always had another life-long struggle which only helped to mask my Acromegaly symptoms—my weight. I was a big baby; I was a pudgy child; and I can't remember a time in my adolescence when I wasn't either trying to lose weight, or stuck in an "in between" period of diet programs. When I was in junior high school, I was probably only about twenty or thirty pounds overweight—this in spite of the fact that I was active in community athletics and school activities. Somewhere between my freshman and sophomore years of high school, though, I started gaining quite a bit of weight, and by the time I graduated high school in 1996, I was morbidly obese. There were so many days I remember being endlessly hungry, even if I had just eaten a feast. I just couldn't seem to control the situation, no matter how hard I tried. Don't get me wrong: I understand personal responsibility. What I couldn't understand was why I was experiencing endless hunger that nobody else seemed to experience. It wasn't just a desire to eat; I was physically hungry. There were so many days when I stopped eating just because I knew I had to—not because I was full. It was so frustrating to know that the feeling of fullness was supposed to be there. It was there for everybody else, but for me, it either wouldn't come or I'd be hungry again shortly after. As time passed, this problem got worse, and my weight seemed to snowball very quickly. How do you go from having twenty or thirty pounds of excess weight to being more than one hundred pounds overweight in just a few years even while remaining active? It was all chalked up to behavior and choice, and I blamed myself over and over again for a situation that I just couldn't figure out how to correct or control.

I never realized that other acromegalics experienced the same appetite frustrations until I joined the Acromegaly Community site just over a year ago. It's not listed as a symptom of Acromegaly in anything that I've ever read, and I have never heard a doctor discuss it as being linked with the condition, not even when I have asked. I have learned over time, though, that doctors are still learning a tremendous amount about Acromegaly. They know what they see and can study—but they can't possibly know what we feel that isn't observable to them. Is every acromegalic obese? No, and I understand that I had this issue long before I had Acromegaly, so I know that Acromegaly wasn't the cause—but I do believe that Acromegaly has significantly exacerbated the problem, beginning in my adolescence.

Speaking of my adolescence, I couldn't possibly discuss this part of my life or journey with Acromegaly without sharing that I was a passionate "band nerd" all through school. "One time at band camp" was a phrase that came out of my mouth long before the *American Pie* movies made it a popular and funny thing to say. I remember wanting to play the clarinet from the time I was six years old and saw a family friend play hers. It was instant love—that glorious black stick with all of those shiny keys making some of the most beautiful and unique sounds I had ever heard. It made some pretty unique sounds when I first started picking it up too, but there wasn't anything glorious about that.

In high school, you don't just play your instrument of choice. You have to wear the twenty-pound polyester band uniform in 100+ degree heat, learn the steps of a show routine on a football field, memorize several pieces of music, march in competitions and parades, and spend hours practicing all of it every day because my school did it to win competitions. I loved it, but it was very time consuming and very exhausting. I always felt like I had to work twice as hard to keep up with the other kids through all of the football games, competitions, and parades. There were some weekends when I slept all day—or both days—as long as we weren't competing. I remember coming home some days after school and just crashing and sleeping through to the next morning. Nobody thought anything of it. I was active. I was a teenager, and teenagers need to sleep a lot. I was also heavier, so my parents just assumed that I wore myself out a bit easier than other kids.

Aside from the sheer exhaustion I felt, there are two things from my "band nerd" days that I remember and, in retrospect, link to Acromegaly. The first is a private music lesson I had where a teacher kept insisting that I needed to make my chin flat and pull it back on the mouthpiece for a better sound instead of letting my chin jut out. No matter how hard I tried during the lesson, I couldn't make my chin flat. It just jutted out beyond what I could control. I didn't remember having that issue in the past, but I remember it being a frustrating issue in that particular lesson. My teacher continuously tried to show me how I needed to form my mouth, and as much as I tried to mimic the exercise, my chin just wouldn't cooperate. When my teacher realized that we were running out of time for the session, he let it go and just told me to be mindful of it and to keep working at it. I did the best I could, but there's only so much control you have over the flexibility of bones. My jaw was growing so much that I was starting to develop an underbite, and I didn't realize it.

The second red flag for Acromegaly that I remember from my "band nerd" days was a pair of shoes. Being a heavier girl, the standard shoes that the other kids ordered from the catalog where all of our band uniforms and accessories came from weren't going to work for me. The shoes didn't come wide enough, and I needed more support for my feet; especially since I was going to be marching so much in the Texas heat. Since the required shoes were a standard white leather, I was able to purchase a pair of shoes more fitting to my needs outside of the catalog. My mom took me to a local shoe company that makes truly wonderful shoes for walking and orthopedics. Admittedly, the store is geared to an older population, but we were able to fit me into a perfect white leather pair of walking shoes, size 8½ WW, and they were like walking on a cloud! I could have cared less who the shoes were designed for. For marching season, they were designed for me, and I bought a new pair every school year. Though I did stay at that shoe size throughout my high school years, thanks to the Acromegaly symptoms, I was not done growing yet. This led to a slightly embarrassing situation for me down the road, which I'll revisit shortly.

After high school, I moved an hour up the road to Austin, Texas, with a group of friends. I went to college part time, supported myself with office work, and enjoyed the newfound freedom of being away from home and doing some fun and stupid things that young adults do. I also learned way too many recipes involving ramen noodles, which I believe is just a rite of passage for people that age. I spent four years in Austin, and just as in high school, I continued to experience days of sleeping and exhaustion for inexplicable reasons. I would occasionally have to call into work because I was just too fatigued to get up and get moving on a particular day. My body seemed almost bi-polar. Some days, I would feel fantastic and be bursting with energy; other days, I would be so sluggish and exhausted I could barely function. I remember the office manager of the company I worked for suggesting some different vitamins and herbs, and I tried just about everything she recommended. I never had much success with her suggestions, but I tried as hard as I could to control my fatigue. After all, who wants their boss pointing out tips on how not to be so exhausted at work? I was young, and I shouldn't have had to worry about this problem. No matter how hard I tried, though, there were just some days where I couldn't hide how exhausted I was: it was frustrating. I have always prided myself on doing well at work, and I didn't want anyone thinking poorly of me in a professional setting. Once again, I just assumed that my weight was to blame, and figured maybe I needed to be more active and to focus more on weight loss. I joined a gym and worked out daily, and I watched what I ate a bit more carefully. With the help and support of my friends and roommates, I did lose a little bit of weight. Unfortunately, even with these positive changes in my lifestyle, I continued to experience the days of exhaustion.

While I was probably one of the biggest kids in my high school, after spending some time as an adult in Austin, I had met several others who struggled with obesity as I had, and I realized there was a major difference between my life and most other obese people I knew. My friends didn't seem to be nearly as fatigued as I was; not even the people I had met who lived a more sedentary lifestyle. Nobody I knew spent an entire day sleeping unless they were sick or went on some kind of party bender. From what I could tell just by spending time with them, they were able to easily keep up with our other peers who were of normal size. A more pro-active and responsible adult probably would have started asking questions about this; but I just wanted to be normal, and I was afraid to get into in depth conversations about some of the things I was experiencing. Maybe they were just built differently than I was, and if only I could lose more weight, I would be able to have that kind of energy too.

Around this time, I also began having menstrual cycles that were very heavy and irregular compared to what I was used to. I had experienced this in high school as well, but in my Austin years (1996–2000), they began to get much worse. I had health insurance through my office job at the time, so I decided to see an OB/GYN to get the issue checked out. This was the first time I had heard of Polycystic Ovarian Syndrome (PCOS). The doctor diagnosed me with this condition in 1998, and it seemed to explain quite a few things. Finally – an answer! The OB/GYN explained that Polycystic Ovarian Syndrome is mainly caused by insulin resistance and is a precursor to diabetes. For the time being, my body was creating enough insulin to keep my blood sugar in check, but my cells weren't responding enough to the insulin to convert the blood sugar properly, so my body continued to produce more insulin. The symptoms for females with this condition include obesity; acne; irregular, heavy or absent menstrual cycles; excess hair (body or facial); male pattern hair loss; infertility; and fatigue. As with most medical conditions, one needn't have all of the symptoms associated to have a confirmed diagnosis. I had most of these symptoms, and I didn't question that I had the condition. I was just relieved to have an answer after all those years.

The relief of the diagnosis didn't last too long though. While it was nice to finally have an answer as to what was causing so many different issues, it wasn't so nice to learn that the treatments for Polycystic Ovarian Syndrome are diet, exercise, possibly Metformin/Glucophage (drugs for diabetes that help with insulin resistance), and birth control. Unfortunately for me, I was only good at the exercise - the rest of the list would be an adjustment for me. I always made an effort to stay active, regardless of my size. Diet was, and still is, a never-ending struggle for me, and since birth control pills are linked with weight gain, I didn't really want to go on them and add to my already intense struggle with weight. I tried the Metformin, but experienced side effects of nausea, headache, and indigestion, so I stopped complying with that part of the treatment. Basically, I had the diagnosis and did very little about the treatment. I went on with life as usual and dealt with the symptoms as best I could.

By spring 2000, I had moved from Austin to Nashua, New Hampshire. One of my closest friends had moved there the previous year, and convinced me to move up after the company I was working for in Austin started to suffer huge financial problems. I was 21, the lease on my apartment was coming up anyway, and I was going to be looking for a new place to live and a new job, so why not throw in a little adventure? I had nothing to lose. I spent a few months doing temporary work in New Hampshire and spending my free time having a blast going for drives in the White Mountains, visiting different beaches in New Hampshire and Maine, and exploring Boston. Then, unexpectedly, my friend who convinced me to go to New Hampshire got an opportunity through his job to go to the New York market, and he decided to take it. I had only been in Nashua a few months, and I wasn't going to stay up there alone, but I didn't want to return to Texas either. I decided to join my friend and make the move to New York with him. I stayed and worked in the city for a few months before my friend and I both ended up in Eastern Long Island with new friends that we had recently met. I realize that sane people don't do these things at random—but who's sane at 21? We had no idea what a bad economy was; you could walk out the door and get a new job any time you wanted. We had both done it again and again. We could have cared less about health insurance; it was just a luxury item we didn't need anyway. We had no idea why Hillary Clinton went around causing all that ruckus a few years back or why she suddenly stopped. We just lived and worked and had as much fun as we could ... and I slept when I needed to.

One of our favorite things to do on Long Island was going out to the outlet store shops in Riverhead. On one of my first trips out there, I thought that my mind was playing tricks on me. There it was! The shoe store where I had gotten my "band nerd" shoes! On Long Island?? How could that be? They were a custom shoemaker that only had stores in San Antonio – or so I thought. I walked over to the store to make sure that it was indeed the same shoe company, and it really was. I don't know how they knew I had moved and that I had missed them the past few years, but I was so glad they leased a store out on Long Island just for me – talk about service! I did a ton of walking in New York, and I couldn't wait to treat my feet to another heavenly pair of their walking shoes.

I'm normally a do-it-yourselfer when it comes to things like pumping gas, parking my car, and buying shoes; but at this store, they like to have their people put the shoes on your feet for you. So, I told the nice sales lady that I took a size 8½ WW in their walking shoe, and she came back with a pair of beautiful, crisp, white walking shoes and a shoe horn. I was giddy at the sight of them. We struck up a nice conversation as she prepared the shoe to put on my foot, but the conversation ceased when she failed to get the shoe on. It didn't fit; it wasn't even close. I looked at her and giggled and said they must just be mislabeled or in the wrong box or something. She suggested getting a larger size, but I had been buying these shoes for years, and I knew exactly what size I wore in them. At my insistence, the sales lady came back with another pair of size 8½ WW walking shoes. She also came back with a pair of size 10WW walking shoes "just in case." Guess what size I ended up buying.

UNBELIEVABLE! FIRST, my favorite local shoe store from Texas opens a location that's not only not in San Antonio, but it's not even in Texas! In fact, it's in the state I would probably consider the polar opposite of Texas! THEN, they change the way they manufacture their shoes and make all of their sizing smaller! What the heck is going on here? I've never been good at keeping my thoughts to myself, so, of course I joked about all of this with the sales lady as she was ringing up my size 10WW walking shoes. Have you ever had someone nervously laugh and smile at you like you're a mental case who's scaring them a little? That poor sales lady! She was older to begin with, and surely never saw young folks going in there and getting excited over their orthopedic shoes. Then, on top of that initial weirdness, she had to deal with someone who was obviously in denial of their shoe size and willing to make up stories about the shoe company changing all of its manufacturing standards to support the denial. No wonder she looked at me like I was a whackadoodle!

I continued to live and work on Long Island through December 2001. I would have liked to stay longer, but the terror attacks sent the local economy (and eventually the national one too) into a bit of a tailspin. Once again, I was working for a company whose days were numbered, and I was struggling to find another job. Additionally, the landlord who owned the house my friends and I were renting together decided to sell it, and I couldn't manage to find another affordable option that was pet friendly. At the time, I had another close friend in the Dallas/Fort Worth area who was about to need a new roommate and could help me find a job. It was a four-hour drive from my family, and I could see them on the weekends. The decision to return to Texas (albeit to another area) was a no brainer. I made the move to Dallas/Fort Worth and started my new job with the sales and catering department of a local hotel there in January of 2002.

When I got settled into my new apartment, I made a trip down to San Antonio for a weekend to see my family. After the initial hugs and excitement of seeing everybody again, I remember my mom staring at my face for the longest time and finally saying, "You look so different. Your face has changed; I guess you must be starting to take on some of the features of your dad's family." This stopped me cold. I had seen it; but I thought I was imagining it. I remembered seeing a photo of myself from a coworker's wedding a few months before I left New York and thinking that it couldn't possibly be my face in the picture—but I knew that it was. I told myself it must have just been a weird angle on the camera. I remembered looking in the mirror and thinking that my nose was bigger and that there was a bit more of a crease at the top where it connected to my brow. I could have sworn that it used to be smooth and flat. In fact, I could have sworn that my whole face used to be relatively flat; but when I turned and looked at a side profile in the mirror, it now looked more like a crescent-moon shape. I didn't even have a double chin anymore, and I had always had a bit of a double chin.

I was silent for a moment while I processed my mother's words and reflected on memories of these incidents and thoughts. I knew exactly what my father's family looked like, and none of them had the facial features that I was developing. Still, to suggest that my nose grew or that my face didn't look the way it was supposed to look was just crazy. This is life; you look the way you look when you age, and you have to accept certain things. Nobody likes getting older, but everybody has to deal with it. The best I knew to tell my mother was that I thought I had seen the changes in my face as well, but I must just be getting older. I think we both knew it had nothing to do with my father's side of the family, but common knowledge said it could only be age or genetics, so she assumed genetics and I assumed age; we were both wrong.

In March 2002, I was struggling to see my computer screen at work, and it was becoming noticeable to my co-workers at the hotel. I also realized that I was battling headaches on a daily basis and took painkillers every day to get rid of them. This was becoming an uncomfortable new routine that I wanted to break. I made an appointment to see the optometrist, assuming that I needed glasses; and I was right—I did need glasses. I had astigmatism in my left eye and was nearsighted in my right, and we corrected this problem in about an hour. It took a few days to adjust to the new glasses, but I did, and went on with life as usual. The headaches didn't stop though, and within a month, I started struggling to see the computer again.

Around this time, I also came down with a urinary tract infection, and needed to go to a general practitioner for antibiotics to clear it up. Fortunately, unlike my jobs in New York, this job did provide me with health benefits. Everybody at my office saw the same doctor who was very close by and came highly recommended, so I thought it was worth checking out. They took me on as a new patient, and we did all of the common workup tests that doctors do with new patients. I discussed the headaches, and during the exam, they found that my blood pressure was slightly elevated. My headaches were low-grade, which they told me was consistent with high blood pressure, so after ruling out the eyeglass prescription, the doctor said that the high blood pressure was probably the cause of the headaches. I was given a prescription to help my blood pressure, antibiotics for the urinary tract infection, and an accu-tester to ensure that the Polycystic Ovarian Syndrome hadn't turned into diabetes. The antibiotics did the trick for the infection; two week's worth of testing had established that I still wasn't a diabetic; and the blood pressure medicine brought my blood pressure into low-normal range. I still had the daily headaches, though.

A few months had passed, and I continued to live, work, and function as normally as I could. It got harder, however, and I couldn't escape the feeling that something was wrong with me. I was tired a lot—more than usual—and the computer at work was getting harder and harder to see. By early August, I had a huge scare. I was driving home from work on the expressway, and suddenly, I was seeing double. It wasn't just double vision, either. It was double vision that wouldn't stay still—kind of like a kaleidoscope. I was dizzy and I thought I would be sick, but most of all, I was scared to death that I was going to get into an accident on the freeway. I hit my head with the palm of my hand repeatedly. I squeezed my eyes open and shut as tightly and rapidly as I could. I couldn't make it stop. I prayed—a lot. I don't remember how I did it, but somehow, I managed to make it home in one piece. When the stress of the incident was over, I walked through my front door, collapsed on the couch, held my little dog, and just cried. I was terrified at what had just happened and decided that I couldn't ignore this.

When I woke up the next day, the double vision was gone, but I was still really freaked out. I called into work and I called the optometrist and told him I needed to see him, that day if possible. Fortunately, he was able to squeeze me in. The testing didn't go too far, though. He gave me a black plastic paddle to cover one eye with while using the other to read the eye chart from left to right. No matter which eye I covered, I could only see half the chart. He asked me if the other half was blurry, and at first, I insisted that there was no other half. All I saw there was black. It wasn't until I lifted the paddle and saw the chart with both eyes that I could see the whole chart from where I was sitting. The optometrist asked me several times if I had hit my head recently, and I told him no (with the exception of trying to correct my double vision the day before). He couldn't help me, but he made an appointment with an ophthalmologist for me within a few days. He told me that if there was something more serious wrong with my eyes, the ophthalmologist should be able to find and treat it after more testing.

It was August 20, 2002. I sat in the waiting room of the ophthalmologist's office and read the material he had on all the various eye diseases people seemed to commonly come in with. I was filled with anxiety as I tried to guess which one of these horrible diseases my eyes had. Would I go blind? Would I have to have surgery on my eyes? People have to be awake for that, don't they? Would it be with a laser or a knife? Would it hurt much? What if they make a mistake when they're cutting and I lose an eye? How long will I be out of work? What if the double vision comes back? Why haven't I told anybody about any of this yet? By the time I got called in, I was nothing but a pile of nerves. Fortunately, the doctor was very calm and reassuring and I was able to relax a bit more as we started the testing.

The testing was only supposed to go for an hour or two in the morning and then I was supposed to go back to work. The doctor told me I needed to call into work for the rest of the day because he needed to dilate my pupils and run more tests than he had originally scheduled me for. I was reluctant to miss any more work, but he made it very clear that my health took priority over my job and I needed to stay. I made the call, let him dilate my pupils, and after waiting for that to take effect, we proceeded with more tests. After several hours, he came to me with various printouts and told me it was the visual field test that told him what he needed to know. The piece of paper he put in front of me showed a print out of two circles, which turned out to be my eyes. Each circle was shaded in half black, half white.

The ophthalmologist explained that the portion in black was where I had completely lost vision in each eye. My jaw dropped and my face contorted in confusion as I tried to process this.

"Are you telling me that I went half blind in both eyes without knowing it?"

"Well, I'm sure you had some signs, but yes, that's what I'm telling you. Your eyes compensate for each other, so unless you have a habit of only looking out of one eye at a time, you wouldn't have realized the severity of the vision loss."

He further explained that the cause of the loss and the double vision was most likely a tumor on the pituitary gland, which was close to the optic chiasm. When the tumors get big enough, they press on the optic nerve, which causes vision loss and double vision, among other things. At least I think that's what he was talking about.

The only thing I heard was *tumor*, and based on his hand gestures, the tumor was in my head. Forget going blind or having eye surgery! I was going to die! That's what happens to people with brain tumors, isn't it? They die! They shave their heads, they go through chemo and radiation, they puke their guts up, and they die. I had gained this vast wealth of knowledge on brain cancer solely through movies, and I had never seen a movie where the brain cancer patient made it. I wondered how long I had and what I would tell my family.

I was on auto-pilot as the ophthalmologist continued to speak to me. He might as well have been the teacher from *Peanuts*. I tried to tune back in, but my mind was racing. The one thing I did manage to pick up on was that he wasn't talking to me as if he had just given me a death sentence. His demeanor was a bit lighter than it should have been in that situation. Something was "off" about that. After a few minutes, I was able to re-engage. I had to figure out why he wasn't speaking in a more serious tone about the situation. Then I heard him utter the word "benign," and I had a completely inappropriate reaction to it. I just burst out with laughter, and it was uncontrollable. It was a Texas college joke I had remembered—"The Aggie's Glossary of Medical Terms." Aggie jokes are equivalent to "redneck" or "blonde" jokes, and anyone who spends a lengthy amount of time in Texas is bound to hear their share of them.

"Benign—what you be after you be eight!" I howled through my laughter.

Tears were running down my face, I was laughing so hard. And you thought the sales lady at the shoe store had it bad! After spending the better part of the day in testing, with the week I had, and the news I had just received, I was one cracked nut! An inappropriate emotional outburst was bound to happen at some point with all of this, but I assume most people would have reacted a bit differently than I did. The man in front of me was a scientist though, and as good natured as he was, he was more interested in discussing what I needed to do next than he was in participating in my pitiful joke.

When I had gotten a grip and pulled myself together, he explained the procedure that they needed to do to get the tumor out, and he told me that I had a really good chance of recovering my vision completely afterward. He called the Medical Center and got me into an MRI within an hour. He also had his receptionist schedule me for an appointment with a neurologist and an endocrinologist the next day. Before I left his office, I remember asking him what would happen if we left the tumor alone. It was a completely nonsensical thing to ask, but the surgery sounded so horrific to me that I wanted the worst case scenario if I decided to do nothing. After all, you should always weigh your options, and it was benign, right? I seriously didn't want to do all that crap the ophthalmologist had just described—it sounded awful! I had stumped him. He just looked at me incredulously and asked why in the world I would choose not to have the surgery. Honestly, in hindsight, I'm surprised he didn't just kick me out of his office. Fortunately, he was very patient with me and explained that not having the surgery wasn't really an option given the size that my tumor must have been at that point. He walked me out to the front desk, and told me to make an appointment with him to re-check my visual fields after I had the surgery. I nodded my head and left his office.

It took me ten minutes to get from the ophthalmologist's office to the radiology department at the nearby hospital. I went through a brief orientation so I would be prepared for what to expect with the MRI, and then before I knew it, I was climbing onto the pull-out table of the machine, being fitted with some headphones, and my head was being locked into a cage to limit movement. I felt like Hannibal Lecter. Then the radiology tech shoved me into the tube. I looked up and saw a thin blue line painted on top of the tube that ran from end to end, and imagined that it was splitting me in half. The rest of the machine was all white, and it surrounded me. I couldn't believe I was there. I prayed that it had all been a bad dream; that there wasn't really a tumor, and I wasn't really in this coffin-like contraption. Tears streamed down my face as I listened to brief directions and explanations from the tech through the headphones. Then the tech asked which radio station I liked, and I was momentarily distracted from all of the fear and negative thoughts as I tried to remember the station number so I could tell her. It took a moment, but I did remember, and gave her the local station I listened to. Within minutes, music was coming through the headphones. I was so grateful for that, and it really did help me to relax a bit for the test. The other small detail that helped me not feel quite so claustrophobic was a small mirror they had attached to the cage on my head. It tilted out so I was able to see my feet and a small area of the room. I had no idea at the time how much of a luxury these two features were, but with all of the MRIs I've had in the years since, this was the only facility I've ever been to that has offered them.

The MRI was very noisy, even with the music. Each portion of it had its own distinct noise, and I felt the vibration of each one. I didn't find the thin blue line or the view of my feet in the mirror tremendously entertaining, so I opted to close my eyes and try to relax as much as possible. In the middle of the testing, the tech came in, pulled me half way out of the tube, and injected contrast dye into my arm. I remember feeling slightly cold at first and then having a metallic taste in my mouth momentarily, but other than that, I didn't have a reaction to it. I was in the tube for a total of about forty-five minutes, and afterward, my head was released from the cage, and I was free to go. I would meet with the neurologist in the morning, and he would have the films and report when I arrived for the appointment.

The drive home was agony. It was rush hour by the time I left the hospital, and there was a ton of traffic on the highway. I was emotionally drained and physically exhausted. I wanted to go home, climb under all of my covers, and hide from the world. I also wanted my mom. I hadn't told her yet, and unfortunately, I was going to have to do it over the phone.

I called, and interrupted a nice dinner out that my mom was having with my stepfather (whom I refer to as "Dad" even though I also have a wonderful relationship with my father – I'm just lucky enough to have two). I didn't want to ruin their evening out, so I told her I would call back in about an hour. She must have heard something in my voice, though, because she insisted that I tell them what I called to tell them then and there. I hesitated for a minute as I tried to figure out the best way to phrase everything, but the effort was futile. The intensity of the day had taken its toll on me, and I just blurted out, "I'm half blind in both eyes and I have a brain tumor." Naturally, I heard silence on the other end of the phone for a minute, and then I heard, "What did you say?" I went on to explain everything I had gone through earlier in the day. Of course, they were upset, and had a million questions, but I didn't have the answers. I was not functioning well at the ophthalmologist's office, so I hadn't retained much of the information he had given me, and I hadn't been on the internet yet to research what a pituitary tumor was. I also still needed to see the kinds of doctors who could give me details. I told my parents that I would keep them posted. Looking back, I still feel a little guilty about how I broke the news to them. They knew nothing about my day to day concerns and the doctor appointments I was scheduling; I never really talked about it with them. Then, suddenly, I called them and dropped a bomb like that in the middle of a pleasant evening out. What were they supposed to do other than worry and feel completely helpless over 250 miles away?

I met with a neurologist first thing the next morning, and he confirmed what the ophthalmologist had told me. There was a large tumor in my pituitary gland, approximately 3.3 cm in diameter, and it had spread into something he was calling the cavernous sinus, which seemed to be of great concern to him. I had no idea what he was talking about, but he brought the MRI films into the room, clipped them to the backlight, and showed me the tumor and cavernous sinus. He explained that the cavernous sinus was where the carotid artery was, and that having a tumor go into that area meant that we knew up front that they would not be able to get the entire tumor out when I had the surgery—it was too dangerous to operate that close to the carotid artery. He continued to do a general neurological exam and was impressed to find that all of my other functions and responses seemed to be normal. He told me that with a tumor that large, there are usually more abnormalities and this was a good sign to him that I should be able to recover my vision after the surgery. He asked if I had an appointment with an endocrinologist, and I confirmed that I had one later that afternoon. He then referred me to a neurosurgeon I would need to work with to have the surgery.

I met with the endocrinologist later the same afternoon, and he really spent quite a bit of time with me. I had no idea how rare my case was, but he did. He primarily specialized in diabetes and thyroid problems, but he took a special interest in my case, and I later learned that he was actually treating another Acromegaly patient who had been diagnosed about three months ahead of me. Looking back, I realize how lucky I was that this doctor took a personal interest in pituitary cases and did a bit of studying to help me and the other patient. In a strange way, we were kind of exciting for him—a break from the norm that he saw coming into his office on a daily basis. The endocrinologist took a very detailed medical history from me and ran just about every test I had ever seen on my blood. His assistant took six tubes! He had suspected Acromegaly from the start, but he also had to rule out other possibilities, and there was one that he couldn't do with my blood. I remember being handed a gallon jug that I had to pee into for a 24 hour period and then return to the lab. This was to rule out a cortisol problem if I remember correctly, and I was absolutely disgusted by it. I know there are worse things, but who wants to tote around a gallon jug of pee for a day? Before leaving the appointment, the endocrinologist told me that he would have the results of the blood work back in a week, and that would tell us what the imbalances were. He told me the treatment would vary depending on what imbalances they found, but that I would most likely be on some kind of medication soon. In the meantime, he would put a call into the neurosurgeon's office to try to expedite my appointment there. Fantastic! Between the optometrist, ophthalmologist, general practitioner, neurologist, endocrinologist, and now the neurosurgeon, I was beginning to feel like a ping-pong ball. That was only the beginning.

Most Americans are at least vaguely familiar with the HIPAA law, and they know that it guarantees your right to privacy with your protected health information. It's unfortunate, but first and foremost, people have to worry about their employment situations, and the effect that their health information can have on their jobs. With the tumor diagnosis, I could now count myself among those who had to consider what information to share with my employer. After all, I had already lost a few days due to all of my recent doctor appointments, and there were more to come. Not only that, but I was about to have brain surgery; that's more than a couple days out of the office due to a cold. I don't know what other people in this situation have shared with their employers, and I know there is not a "one size fits all" solution, but I decided the best route for me to take would be the "full enchilada." I was working with a great group of people who valued me and my work, and we were as much of a "family" as a professional group of people could be. I knew that being up front with them and explaining the situation in its entirety would be the best option, and having the conversation with my director was the very first thing I did upon my return to the office. Fortunately, I was right, and she and the team were very supportive and worked with me to allow more flexibility in my schedule for the increase in doctor appointments we knew were coming. They even went a step further and took up a small collection to help me with the co-pays. To this day, I still consider them the best group of people I have ever had the pleasure of working with.

Over the next few weeks, the doctor appointments continued to pile up. There were initial appointments, follow-up appointments, and more referrals. The neurosurgeon had to refer me to an ear, nose, and throat (ENT) doctor because that doctor would be working with him to perform the incision and suturing under my lip and nose for the surgery. I had to do a CT scan for this doctor as the MRI apparently didn't show him what he needed. Fortunately, the CT machine was big and open, and the test was much faster than the MRI had been. After the neurosurgeon and ear, nose, and throat doctor had collaborated on my tests and their schedules, they set a surgery date for me in mid-September. In the meantime, the endocrinologist had confirmed that I did indeed have Acromegaly, and my IGF-1 levels were 1181; normal range shouldn't have put me past 250 on that scale if I remember correctly, so this was definitely an extreme imbalance. He referred me to a cardiologist to check up on the condition of my heart, and also to ensure that I was fit for surgery—another battery of tests. He also referred me to a gastroenterologist to have a colonoscopy, as Acromegaly is known to be a risk factor for colon cancer. He told me I could do that one after the surgery though, as he knew I was already overwhelmed with everything going on. He also started me on three daily injections of a medication to shrink the tumor before surgery, and to help control the IGF-1 levels; there was an appointment to learn how to administer the injections for that as well.

My life seemed to revolve more around hospitals and doctor appointments than work, friends, and fun for that time period. I was worn out; I was afraid of having the surgery; I was depressed; I got sick to my stomach and had to lay down every time I injected what I viewed as poison into my body; and for the first time ever, I was truly jealous of my friends. I had their youth, but I envied their health. I resented that they didn't have to go through what I was going through. They could go to work and school and go out and do all the normal things that people our age did without a care in the world—or at least without a care of anything more serious than failing a class or getting in trouble at work. I had to make myself sick three times a day with those horrible injections, and I was about to have brain surgery. I was afraid that I might not wake up from it, or that something else might go wrong. As supportive as they were trying to be, they had no idea what this felt like; how much it pained me just to watch them run around and do all of the things they did and take life for granted like we had always done in the past. I'm not usually a jealous person, and I've always tried to be thankful for what I have in life; but during this time period, I was anything but thankful. I tried to hide it as best I could; nobody wants to be around someone who is miserable all the time, and I needed their support in spite of how I was feeling.

One of my closest friends had a bit more freedom in his schedule, and he was able to accompany me on several of my doctor appointments leading up to my surgery. I don't remember how appreciative I was about it then, but his being there with me was invaluable and helped make the drudgery of the doctor appointments much more tolerable. He is definitely my "goof off" partner in life, and he can bring fun to nearly any situation. I'm sure we were annoying to other patients and medical staff during the times we were at the appointments together, but I needed the release that the goofing off and laughter brought to such a serious situation. I remember sitting in the neurosurgeon's office with my MRI films and looking around at all of the other patients with their MRI films; we would make up funny stories about what we thought was wrong with everybody else and how they got whatever injury or illness they were in there for. When we went into exam rooms, my friend would go through all of the drawers and pull out whatever equipment was in there and start playing with it. The less he knew about the instrument, the funnier it was to watch him try to figure out what to do with it—especially when a doctor or nurse walked in on us in the process. We would both listen to what a doctor had to say intently, and then before I could think of a real question to ask, my friend would sometimes ask a ridiculous one, which caused the two of us to crack up in front of a doctor who rarely seemed to appreciate the humor as much as we did. Whoever said "Laughter is the best medicine" was onto something. Well, I can't truly say that it's the best medicine because a laughing spell won't kill a tumor; but it sure does help make the medicine a lot more tolerable.

In the week leading up to my surgery, I had made every arrangement I could think of. I had done plenty of online research and found a pituitary tumor group online to chat with about the surgery; I had applied and been approved for my short term disability benefits through work; I had given my office the dates I would be out and arranged for my friend to temp part-time in my place for them as he had previously worked there and had a bit of availability with his schedule; I had toured the ICU of the hospital and met with the staff there to be given an overview of what to expect after I came out of surgery; I had completed a living will and given my family information about my assets, debts and how the life insurance was to be split in the unlikely event of my death; I had made room for my parents to stay at my place for the surgery and written directions down to the various places they would need to get to in the area; and most importantly, I had psychologically readied myself to the best of my ability. I had made peace with going in for the surgery and all of the possible results. I didn't know that I was about to hit one more major snag two days prior to my surgery date—the pre-surgery blood work.

If my memory serves correctly, it is standard for doctors to take pre-surgery blood work 24 hours before a patient goes under. One of the things they test for is something called a PTT. The long words that this acronym stand for aren't as important as knowing what it means. Basically, it's a test doctors run to see how quickly your blood clots. For some surgeries, your blood may clot too quickly, and a doctor may need to give an anti-coagulant to slow this process down. In other cases, your blood may not clot quickly enough, and a doctor will be concerned that you could bleed out during surgery. In my case, it was the latter. The neurosurgeon's assistant called me the day before my surgery and let me know that I couldn't have my surgery the next day because my PTT was abnormal. I felt my stomach drop as if I had just gone down the steepest hill of a roller coaster. What did that mean? Now something's wrong with my blood? What do I have to do now? When would I be having the surgery? I'm already scheduled out of work! My parents are driving up from San Antonio RIGHT NOW! There wasn't anything the assistant could do but apologize and refer me to a hematologist, whom they had scheduled me with the next morning. How swell! I didn't have enough doctors in my life, so let's add another to the pile! At this point, I had quit smoking over a year ago – a nasty habit I had from my senior year in high school until August of 2001, and I truly never looked back after I had gotten it out of my system. The day the neurosurgeon's assistant called and told me I couldn't have the surgery the next day as planned, I fought the urge to smoke harder than I ever remember fighting it the day after I quit.

My mom accompanied me to the hematologist appointment the next day where more blood was drawn for more tests. We met with the hematologist briefly to discuss the possibilities for the abnormal PTT, and my mom shared with him that it could be a genetic trait that she was aware of on her side of the family. She explained that while they weren't hemophiliacs (people who easily bleed and whose blood doesn't easily clot), there was a lower fibrinogen (clotting agent in blood) level that runs on her side of the family. The hematologist did confirm that a low fibrinogen level would cause an abnormality in the PTT, and he said it was one of the things they would be testing for. My mom just looked at me and said she was so sorry I was going through all of this, and that she hadn't thought of this particular issue sooner. I didn't blame her at all; with everything she had going on, how was she supposed to anticipate something like that? I was just grateful to have her there. The hematologist told us he would have the results of the test the next day and would call to tell us what I needed to do next. When his call came, it was to confirm what my mother had told him: that I also had the low fibrinogen count, and that I would need to have a blood transfusion before my surgery to ensure that I didn't bleed out. The neurosurgeon had apparently also been in contact with the hematologist because I received a call from his assistant later in the day to advise me of my new surgery date: October 7, 2002.

I couldn't afford to stay out of work for the next few weeks on short term disability, so I had to undo a few of those arrangements until it was time to go back in. Once again, the team of people I worked with were completely supportive and understanding and accommodated the schedule change, as did my friend and the short term disability company. My parents also adjusted the time off they had arranged for as well, and once again, I had to go through the whole process of psyching myself up for the surgery. Sometimes I think the medical community at large is just so used to dealing with major medical issues on a day-to-day basis that they don't quite realize all of the things people have to do to get ready for major treatments. The psychological trauma that comes about as a result of these events is impossible to describe to those who haven't experienced it for themselves. I was beginning to understand why old people talk about their surgeries and medical conditions so much. It was a battle; something gut-wrenching and scarring (physically and emotionally) that they had survived and lived to tell about. When I came to this realization, I decided that I hoped to one day be an old person myself who got to bore the hell out of younger people by talking about mine.

The night before my surgery, my parents accompanied me to the hospital, got me checked in, sat with me while I had the blood transfusion, and left when visiting hours were over. They would be back first thing in the morning before I went under anesthesia for the surgery. I don't remember much more about that night, other than that I didn't sleep well, which was to be expected given the situation. The next morning, there was a flurry of activity around me as a group of people came in filling a variety of different roles to get me ready for the surgery. I remember climbing onto a rolling bed, having a blue hair cap put on me, and kissing my parents goodbye as I was wheeled away. I prayed that it wouldn't be the last time I would get to see them. I had one IV in my arm as I climbed onto the table in the operating room. The anesthesiologist was in there along with the ear, nose, and throat doctor, the neurosurgeon, and a group of other people I had never seen before. They were talking in medical language, and I understood very little of what they were saying. I didn't really need to; within seconds, the anesthesiologist put the mask on my face, and told me to count down backward from ten. I'm not sure what number I made it to, but I went away for the length of time that these people were digging around in my head.

In spite of my pre-surgery prayers, I woke up wishing I had died during the surgery. My face hurt like crazy; I had a massive headache; and I was heaving to throw up because the anesthesia had made me sick to my stomach. I had boot pumps on my legs, a catheter coming out my great below, a tangle of tubes connected to IV's in both arms, an oxygen monitor on my finger, and a morphine pump in my right hand. I had an incision in my lower abdomen where the neurosurgeon had taken some fat to help seal my nose (or at least I think that's what he said he was going to do with it); tape over an area near my neck where they had tried and failed to run a central line; and a team of people who all seemed to be trying to talk to me at once. One of them took my cap off and mentioned how beautiful my thick, curly brown hair was. If I hadn't been heaving, I probably would have shouted expletives at her. I felt anything and everything but beautiful at that moment. Someone had pushed anti-nausea medication into my IV and the nausea and heaving almost instantly came to a halt, but the pain and discomfort just couldn't be abated. I pressed the morphine pump like crazy once I knew what it was; anything to get out of the pain. Unconsciousness was the only relief there would be for days. When I woke up on occasion and could bear being conscious for a while, I realized I felt dizzy and sick again and I had to close my eyes. From what I could tell, I had completely recovered my vision, and it was so overwhelming to visually take in all of the light and activity around me that it made me sick.

I think it was 24 hours before I was able to eat or drink anything, but my mouth was seriously dry and felt so gross. I remember there being some sponges on sticks that were dipped in a mint liquid of some kind, and it helped to rub them on my lips and to be able to suck on them for a little bit. Medical staff of one kind or another came in to do different things to me at least once an hour, it seemed. The morning following my surgery, they decided to take me on a trip down to the MRI machine to take a look at my pituitary post-op. If I thought the MRI was unpleasant prior to surgery, it was REALLY unpleasant when I was recovering from surgery. I got through it though, and it was determined that the surgery was a success; there was no evidence of the tumor anywhere but in the cavernous sinus. I knew I was far from being out of the woods, but it was a piece of good news, and I was thrilled to hear it; or at least I would have been if I could have thought of anything other than the desire to be unconscious again.

I was in the hospital for a total of five days. I spent three days in the ICU and two more on the regular floor. There wasn't anything particularly wrong to keep me in the ICU for three days; they just didn't have room for me on the regular floor by the time I should have been moved from the ICU. This was the first time I had ever had surgery of any kind, and I remember so many things happening over those few days. Mostly, aside from the intense discomfort, I remember the feeling of complete helplessness that I had never experienced before. There wasn't a single part of my body that wasn't connected to something, and I couldn't have moved much if I wanted to. Any sense of modesty I may have had was out the window. Attendants came in with wet bathing cloths to wipe me down once or twice a day and to look at various parts of my body to ensure everything was clean, not developing infection, and functioning properly. I remember doctors and medical students that had nothing to do with my case coming in to see me, and my mother getting fed up and telling them to leave. I remember looking forward to seeing one nurse in particular every evening because he talked to me like I was a real person instead of just another patient lying in a bed. When you're in that kind of situation, you can very easily lose any sense of your dignity and humanity, and anybody who gives you a hint of normalcy is more valuable than all the gold in the world. I remember feeling somewhat energetic and normal one day and then fatigued and sleeping through most of the next, and I remember how my mind betrayed me when I was finally ready to get out of bed and start walking. I mistakenly thought I could just get up and do that like I always had, but after four days of lying in a hospital bed, I would have gone straight down if it weren't for the help of a nurse and my mother. And then there was the nasal packing; how could I forget? Shortly before I checked out of the hospital, they took out the nasal packing, and it was like a magic trick! The string of cotton just continued to come out - did they seriously get all of that up my nose? I had no idea there was that much room up there!

As far as complications go, I was fairly lucky. I didn't have a spinal fluid leak, I hadn't developed any infections, and the pain seemed to become more bearable after a couple of days. In fact, I had to switch from morphine to Demerol by the third day because the morphine was giving me a huge headache; and I was only on Demerol for a day before switching to Vicodin. The only complication I did develop was diabetes insipidus, which is a condition where the kidneys can't conserve water, and it is common and usually temporary after pituitary surgery. It only lasted about a week for me. Overall, aside from the first couple days of pure misery post-op, I had a pretty good recovery, and after I had left the hospital, I felt completely normal after about three weeks. Of course, there were still post op appointments, but in time, these would die down.

With the surgery behind me, I had gone back to the ophthalmologist to confirm that I had completely recovered my vision, and after another few hours of testing with him, he was happy to report that I had. I didn't really need him to tell me that, but it seemed important to have it documented in my medical records. I also got in contact with the gastroenterologist to set up the colonoscopy. It was really pretty standard. The night before was disgusting with drinking a large amount of a thick, clear liquid for the purpose of getting "cleaned out." Then, the next morning, my mom took me to the hospital. I checked in, they put an IV in me, knocked me out, and when I woke up, I was appalled that someone in the room was letting out the most obnoxiously loud farts I had ever heard. They weren't saying "excuse me" or anything! Then I realized I was the only one in the room. A nurse came in, and I was so embarrassed; I couldn't control it! She just told me it was natural and I needed to let it out because they had "aired up" my colon for the procedure, and my body had to get rid of it. No problem there! I was a farting machine for a good 30 minutes! God bless nurses! I have no idea why anybody would sign up for that job! They released me, and I had a pretty normal day after that. I can't say it was a pleasant experience, but it was far from the worst I had been through. The results were back within a week, and everything was normal. Given my age, I wouldn't have to have another one for 7-10 years.

The next thing I had to focus on was the hormones; if only that were as simple as the colonoscopy was. Every pituitary surgery patient runs the risk of losing pituitary function, so we had to rule that out. Fortunately, my tests concluded that my pituitary was functioning normally. We also had a small hope that my IGF-1 levels would normalize after surgery, as all acromegalics do; but that just wasn't the case for me. They were in the 700 range with no medication, which is a big improvement from 1181, but still nowhere near normal. The endocrinologist started me on monthly injections to control the tumor and side effects, which still made me feel cruddy for the first week, but I was so grateful to only have to do it once a month instead of three times a day. It helped, but over time, it stopped being effective and he increased the dose. Once again, it helped but never brought my levels into normal range. This was during the time when an alternative was still in trials, so the original shot was the only drug available aside from the earlier pill medications that were not easily tolerated and not quite as effective from what I was told. Within a year though, the other drug became available and I was switched from one monthly injection to one daily injection of the new medication. I wasn't thrilled about that, but I was grateful that the new drug didn't produce any noticeable side effects, and I seemed to feel better on it. In time though, we had learned that even the new drug didn't normalize my levels. Next, we went for a combination treatment of both drugs, and that was not fun at all. I always had to see doctors to have the monthly injection. It was inconvenient and never pleasant as the needle was so large. Then I had to continue giving myself daily injections, but that was only on the months where I could actually get both drugs. The evils of the U.S. health care system had finally hit me with my Acromegaly diagnosis.

About a month after the surgery, I had received bills from every kind of medical group that had a staff member walk into the room, whether I had ever heard of them or not. Insurance only covered so much, after all. I paid what I could, but mostly, I let them fall into collections, ensuring that I took care of the doctors I would need to continue to see over and over again. It's a terrible choice to have to make, but it was the only option I had. Then there were the drugs. Because both shots are specialty drugs, and very expensive ones at that, the insurance company required what's called a pre-authorization. Every month, the pre-authorization had to be put into their system, and every month, it was a battle. As most insurance companies do, my insurance company at the time decided to split their pharmaceutical and medical operations and have a subcontracted prescription benefit manager run their pharmaceutical benefits. I would call the insurance help line, and they would tell me that my pre-authorization for prescriptions didn't fall under them, and that I had to go through the prescription benefit manager. I would then call the prescription benefit manager and be told that because the drugs were specialty injectibles, they fell under the medical part of the plan and I would have to call the regular health insurance help line—the one I had just called. I would have to get a letter from my endocrinologist's office every time the pre-authorization expired, and I couldn't get help from either help line. Eventually, I had to have my company's corporate HR contact the plan to have this situation resolved, and it took some time for them to change it. When they did, they simply extended the period of time that the pre-authorization was in the system, and after a few months, it would expire again, and I would go through the process again. It was exhausting. This was when I realized that the best thing I could do in the eyes of an insurance company was to die, and they were more than willing to help make that happen by denying the very benefits my employer and I paid them to cover. I've hated them ever since.

In January 2005, in hopes of eventually being able to come off all of the drug therapies, I decided to have radiation. There was a facility in San Antonio that was offering a newer, more precise method of radiation called Cyber Knife, and it seemed like a good option considering how small and delicate the area of the cavernous sinus is. The preparation for this procedure involved making some strange kind of mask for my face and a more contrasted MRI. The mask was no big deal, but the MRI used a machine they called a "power injector" if I remember correctly. Was it ever! I had to have an IV placed in my arm prior to the MRI rather than a tech coming in and just injecting contrast in the middle of my MRI. When it was time for the injection of contrast, the machine shot that stuff through my veins so fast that I started feeling nauseous and like I was going to pass out or just die right there. I don't remember ever having that feeling before or since, but I'll never forget it. I recovered within about ten minutes, but it was the scariest thing while it was happening. I don't think I'll be agreeing to let anyone hook me up to a "power injector" again. That kind of terminology should be used for cars, not people.

After my tests had been reviewed by the radiation oncologist and his team, he had established that I would need three sessions with a specified dosage to deliver the total dosage he thought I would need. Within a week of the prep work we had done, I went in, laid down on a table, was fitted with the very same mask they had made from my head, and a huge robotic arm moved all around me shooting radiation into my head from various angles. It felt like something you would see in a science fiction movie where someone gets abducted by aliens. After the procedure, I was given a prescription for a steroid to reduce any swelling in my head, and my mom and I went home expecting to return the day after next for the second treatment.

Recovery from the radiation was horrible. I was fatigued and exhausted from the radiation and had to stay in bed most of the time; but the steroid I was on to reduce the brain swelling kept me from being able to sleep. It also made me insanely hungry. I had been on it after my tumor surgery as well, and I remember the hunger it caused, but I guess since I was also taking Vicodin at the time, it didn't cause such a disruption in being able to sleep. I was miserable. The day after my treatment, the radiation oncologist told me not to come in for the second treatment. There was a concern about the calibration of the machine, and he believed I may have been given more radiation in the initial dose than they had planned. He would let me know about the third treatment in the next day or so. I was confused and angry. I wondered if I would have felt as bad if I had been given the lower dose of radiation. I wondered if a week out of work was truly enough time to recover given how badly I felt. Another day had passed and I received another call from the oncologist telling me that he thought it would be best if I didn't come back for another treatment. He explained that I didn't receive all of the radiation I was supposed to have received, but I received more than he wanted to add on to at that point. He thought the radiation I did receive was more than enough to see some results, and that the best thing to do was to give it time. After my experience, I certainly wasn't anxious to jump back up on that table, so I was upset and frustrated and felt horrible, but I decided I was done with this option. I've had a few people who have heard this story ask me why I never thought of suing this doctor for not ensuring that the machine was calibrated properly, thus giving me a "botched" radiation job. My answer to this is fairly simple; I do not believe in frivolous lawsuits. This doctor and his team were trying to help me, and in the process, made a mistake. The mistake resulted in a few days of unpleasantness for me, but they didn't deliver more radiation than I was supposed to receive overall, and nothing they did caused irreparable harm. I recovered and I went back to work. I believe medical lawsuits are only called for when the mistake a physician makes results in loss of life, limb or functionality of some kind that impairs an individual's ability to live and work normally; or that results in additional medical costs that need to be covered. Fortunately, that wasn't the case for my radiation treatment, and I just wanted to get on with my life.

It's been over five years now since I had that procedure, and there has been no change in my IGF-1 levels as a result of it. If the radiation helped with anything, it seems to have prohibited the growth of new tumor cells in my pituitary and cavernous sinus. Every MRI I have had since has shown nothing visible but scar tissue, so

I suppose if it at least kept the tumor from re-growing, it was worth doing. Sadly though, I remain dependent on medications, which is a disappointment considering the reason I opted for radiation to begin with. I believe in later years, it was determined that Cyber Knife was not as effective as Gamma Knife, which leaves me to wonder how different my outcomes might have been if I had opted for the Gamma Knife instead. I suppose I'll never know.

I made a move from Dallas/Fort Worth to San Antonio in September of 2005, another move to New York City in October of 2007, and another move to the Hudson Valley in February 2010. It's likely that I'll be returning to San Antonio again soon or possibly starting a new adventure somewhere else. It's how I live my life; it's what I do. At some point, I'm sure I'll settle, but for now, this is how I live. With each new city I go to, I ensure that I have health insurance through COBRA until I can get on a new employer's plan, and I always ensure that the jobs I take actually have decent plans I can depend on (as best as insurance can be depended upon anyway). I establish myself with local doctors and the best endocrinologists I can find. If they don't have a working knowledge of Acromegaly and are willing to invest themselves, I will work with them. I haven't found a doctor yet who wasn't interested in my case. At this stage in the game, I've had the surgery and radiation, so all that's left is testing for IGF-1 levels, an annual MRI, and prescribing medications. I can work with nearly any doctor on doing that as long as I stay diligent on the studies going on and see about new options for treatments that I may want to try. I remain hopeful in this area as I've seen the release of new drug alternatives into the market from the time I was diagnosed and am currently aware of trials for an implant drug. For a rare disease, that's a lot of advancement to come out in eight years! When you're undergoing the initial surgery or some kind of major treatment like radiation, it's hard not to let the disease run your life and your thoughts—but in the long run, you get to have most of your days and live almost normally. There are good days and bad days. Some days, I'm just exhausted and need to sleep, and I'll have other various symptoms as well. I know that those are a result of the disease. But I have a lot of normal days and even some days where I feel great too, and I'm thankful for each and every one of them. I do the best I can to ensure that this disease doesn't run my life, while making sure that I'm responsible enough to make certain accommodations for myself because I have it.

I also have tried to be a bit more active in the online community as I've recently realized how big and organized it has become. I'm truly amazed at all of the people with this condition who have come together to support each other and the newly diagnosed. I have hope that in the future, we'll see many more advancements and be able to help people catch this disease earlier so they can be spared the long paths and treatments that quite a few of us with this disease have had to take. I assume anyone who is reading this has either been newly diagnosed or has a loved one who has been. You have been through or seen all of the frustrating symptoms and mysteries leading up to diagnosis and are now potentially facing some really scary treatments. I'm sure you'll experience every emotion possible of a human being, and that's to be expected. My hope though, is that throughout the journey you're about to embark on, you will keep your humor and will remain hopeful. Just remember that so many of us have been through this and survived, and we're here to talk to; and there are people in the world working on advancements in treatment for this disease all the time. It's been eight years, and I still have difficulty with my IGF-1 levels, but I remain hopeful that this will not always be the case for me; and for the days where I'm frustrated and not feeling so great, I have friends online I can talk to who know EXACTLY what I'm going through.

Danielle Roberts is an administrative professional and aspiring writer. She currently resides in San Antonio, TX, where she is pursuing a degree in English. Her struggles with Acromegaly and seeking affordable care through private insurance in the U.S. health care system helped her to develop a passion for health care in politics and for the struggles of others in seeking the care they need. She uses her experience in working for non-profit medical organizations as well as her personal experiences to reach out to others struggling with health concerns, and to help them navigate their options whenever possible.

She continues to learn and navigate her own treatment options in an ever-changing health care system, and remains hopeful for more effective and affordable treatment options for Acromegaly and other difficult health conditions in the future.

Fear and the Disease: Acrophobia

Michael Cookman

You can conquer almost any fear if you will only make up your mind to do so. For remember, fear doesn't exist anywhere except in the mind.

—Dale Carnegie

When you go to the doctor because of an ear problem, you expect to hear that it's no big deal, we can take care of that right now. You don't expect to be told you have, say, a tumor in your brain. But that's just what happened when I went to see a primary care physician for the first time since I was a child.

My right ear had been fading a little, and I could not hear as well on that side as on the other; so I made an appointment with a doctor who I learned was one of five I could see, according to my insurance plan at work. I'd never had to choose a doctor before. I thought you just went to see whatever doctor was near home and that was that.

The doctor I went to see about the hearing trouble is Dr. C.

Dr. C's office was part of St. Francis Hospital in Evanston, Illinois. This worked out well because it was not far from where I lived, just a few stops on the L train line, and it was a nice little walk from the train to the hospital and then to her office. I had to fill out some forms, but from then to being called to see her was just a couple of minutes. I told her about my hearing troubles, and she asked me if I had ever heard of Acromegaly.

"Acromegaly? No, I'm pretty sure I've never heard of that. Is it a new rock band?"

She did not fall on the floor laughing as I had hoped, but she did smile and say, "Well, no. It's an illness where your pituitary gland produces too much growth hormone."

Oh. Well, that didn't sound too serious, I thought. How bad can too much of that be? I asked if there was a medication that one takes for such a thing, and she said, "Well, sort of."

The way she said that made me feel, this might be something worth thinking about. After she cleaned my ear, she suggested I go to a different portion of the hospital and get an MRI done on my brain, which is where the pituitary is situated. So I made an appointment for the following week.

I went on about life as usual, going to work at the bookstore I've been with for more than ten years and doing my weekly magic show at a local coffee shop a block from my apartment in Chicago's Rogers Park, North Side. The coffee shop is the place where I also met my girlfriend Sal (Girlfriend? Lady friend? What do you say when you're 40 years old? I'm going to say girlfriend. You don't like it, think of something else) when we were both regulars, and fate and/or destiny brought us together. But I'm getting a little ahead of myself. So . . .

. . . Actually things were getting kind of dull, and I was looking to make some changes: do more with my life than just work at the store and go home and read, go out for drinks with co-workers and whoever else tagged along. I did do the occasional kids show at a grade school in the city, but that didn't really count as something on the regular agenda, though I did rehearse a lot.

What I was looking for, I do not know. What changed my life, I did not see coming.

I knew there was something wrong with my pituitary gland, but I didn't think that could be serious, mostly because I didn't know what this gland was, or even where it was. I had heard of it, sure, but I thought it was something like your tonsils, and when something happens to them, you have them removed and you eat a lot of ice cream.

I arrived at the hospital about a half hour before my appointment. I figured there would be a lot of people waiting around, and I knew there would be paperwork. Best to always plan ahead. Much to my surprise, there was nobody there except the nice lady behind a desk with a computer and a bunch of files. She already knew who I was and gave me the forms to fill out and said it would just be a few minutes, and I glanced at her typewriter and saw a form with my name and the words POSSIBLE BRAIN TUMOR; and that's when I knew this could be serious. It's a good thing she told me to be seated because I might have fainted at this news; I know that my legs definitely felt weak. I filled out the forms and comforted myself with the notion that I had looked at the wrong form, it must be somebody else. Then she handed me that form, and I knew the fix was in, so to speak.

Here I was in an office for an MRI, and I didn't even know what that was, but I would learn it stood for magnetic resonance imaging, which sounds a lot cooler. The nice lady escorted me to another room with lockers, and I had to change into a hospital gown and leave everything in one of the lockers, especially keys and anything else magnetic. All I kept thinking was, what have I gotten myself into here? I'll tell you what: a day in the MRI machine can be summed up as being in a big, scary machine that makes unfriendly noises and has a conveyor belt you lie down on, but you need earplugs in your ears (of all places) before you ride backwards into the machine where suddenly your whole world is about two inches on either side of your vision, and you can't move or everybody will have a bad day. So for everyone to be happy, I had to have a very scary day!

The machine makes a series of clanging sounds like someone is trying to get inside your tin can, and then after a couple of minutes it just stops. Two or three more minutes and it starts up again, and this goes on for about a half hour. Then the conveyor belt politely rolls you out, and you have never been more happy to be able to move again. Bonus: you get to put your clothes on and go home.

At work everyone said I was going to be fine, that this was all just routine and not to worry. That's nice of them, but thinking about the possibility of having a tumor in your brain overrides polite people telling you it's all okay.

The results of the MRI would be available in about a week, so after about a million years I got a call from Dr. C, and she told me I definitely have a brain tumor and something needs to be done about this, so I went to see her and learn about my options. It's a pleasant little walk from the L train in Chicago through a nice neighborhood of houses and apartments, and it was a nice, quiet autumn morning as I went strolling toward the hospital with plenty of time to worry.

A tumor? What the hell is a tumor? And why is it there? Am I going to have seizures now, am I going to melt, will I still be able to see the colors of the rainbow? Why can't I just have narcolepsy? At least you get some sleep that way.

Inside Dr. C's office she explained to me that this tumor produces too much growth hormone and that's why my forehead and jaw are so pronounced—not that I noticed, but she certainly did. She asked me whether I had noticed any changes over the years. I didn't much like the way my hands were kind of swelling at the knuckles, and my teeth were getting weird—kind of separating. And speaking clearly had become an issue. But I thought these things just happened to everybody upon advancing years, and I've always considered myself very ordinary, certainly not the kind of person that gets weird illnesses.

Well, as it happened, I was wrong. All of these things were signs of Acromegaly and were the result of this tumor in my brain. Not on my foot, or arm, no. In my brain.

Dr. C set me up with an appointment to see a surgeon who operates on people with this Acromegaly, and as rare as it is, I wondered how much experience a surgeon could have operating on this sort of thing. I was reasonable, though, since I knew I sure couldn't do it myself.

The surgeon's name is also C, and so as not to be too confusing, let's call him Dr. Ct. His office was a bit farther away, in Skokie, a short trip from the city of Chicago. When I walked in, it was I expected in the beginning of my medical journey. This looked pretty much like every other doctor's office: a small waiting room with three or four other patients all looking over magazines or at the floor or whatever else they can do to not look at each other. After a few minutes of me wondering if this was some big, elaborate joke someone was playing on me, an employee walked me to an office and said the doctor would be in shortly.

Shortly after that, Dr. Ct came in, and at first I thought he was the young apprentice they often send in for preliminary questions; but this was the surgeon himself. He appeared to be about twelve years old with short, closely cut brown hair and a smiley Brady Bunch face. He put my MRI photos (x-rays, whatever) on a thing on the wall and proceeded to tell me about the tumor.

All I could understand was that it was there and it had to come out. And that if it didn't come out sometime soon, I could go blind, lose various functions I would prefer to keep, and/or die before my time. That's an expression I've never completely understood. Who knows when the right time to die is? If I die by getting hit by a car tomorrow, how do I know it was before my time? Maybe it was after my time? Or maybe I don't have a time; maybe I get to die any time I want to. Anyway, I understood it was serious, and I agreed to have the surgery in two weeks from that date. And that gave me plenty of time to worry and feel sorry for myself.

So that's why my hands looked kind of twisted and my head was taking on a different size around the temples. All because of this tumor—whatever that was—inside of my brain. I didn't want to have a tumor. I didn't get sick hardly at all; in fact the only notable time was when I was a kid and I had bronchitis, but that was a small price to pay to get out of school for a couple of days. My mom was scared as can be about this bronchitis, but I got over it soon enough and that was that.

But this Acromegaly. Jeez. Takes a long time just to be able to say it; imagine explaining it to people, especially when you don't know much about it yourself. Well-meaning friends automatically think they become experts all of a sudden, telling you that the doctors are all wrong and there's no such thing as a pituitary tumor and "if this then that" and "if that then this"; and I decided I would go with what the doctors said, since they are trying to help me too, and have the medical background to back up their opinions.

Surgery was scheduled for a Monday morning, and the previous Sunday I spent most of the day home alone, and scared. The surgery could go wrong and I could wake up blind, or it could go even more wrong and I could wake up dead, and then I'd really be depressed. Or it could go well and I'd be cured. Still, there was a tumor in my brain, and I didn't want it there or anywhere else for that matter. This was the first time I'd ever had to think about my own mortality, and I kept thinking things like I would not be here next Christmas or any other holiday and I would never see my sister or brother or cousins again.

I decided I didn't want to think that way and took my guitar and a blanket down to the lake where I sat on the grass and played for a while—until clouds hurried in and started raining. I took that as a sign that I was being overly melodramatic, so I headed on home.

Monday morning at 4:00 a.m. was dark; and as I walked to the L train near home, lightning flashed all over, not just in the sky but on the buildings and on the sidewalk and in my eyes, and I wondered if it was trying to get to me before the surgeon. Then I smiled at the thought. It felt good to smile, and I realized I hadn't done so for some time. I wanted to make sure the smile wouldn't be wasted, so I looked into a window of one of the local stores to see my smiling face with the lightning flashing just in time, so I could get a good view. Then I remembered I had not brushed my teeth and hoped that wouldn't bother the doctors later on.

The L train was nearly empty. The only other people were sleeping with their heads resting on the backs of the seats in front of them, and there were plenty of empty seats. I didn't sit down though. I was only going three stops and I was a little keyed up anyway. We got to my stop at South Boulevard, and the lightning was keeping the area bright as I walked the four blocks to the hospital. I was back to being scared again.

My hospital room was tiny. Just the one bed, on which two little, young nurse apprentices told me to lie down, and they asked me if I needed anything, all happy and chirpy and ready for anything. I told them I could use a new life, and they laughed (I think) and said if they could, they would. They vanished behind a door, and I was alone for a couple of minutes. Then a big bodybuilder of an orderly came in and said we were now going to the operating room, and he grabbed the metal railing of the bed and yanked both me and the bed forward toward the door. I just hoped he wasn't going to slug me. But then, we were in a hospital, so what difference would it make?

I had envisioned the journey to the operating room as a ride down a long, spacious corridor lined with a choir on both sides singing hymns. Then huge, tall doors would part, and an audience would applaud your entrance, and a French horn would sound a majestic tune, and dancing girls would sing, "Welcome to surgery." Alas, this was not the case. The orderly dragged me ten feet across the hall and pushed open a door with the bed, and a handful of doctors stood around, one of whom was the twelve year old guy I'd interviewed with a couple weeks ago.

"Hey, guy!" he said. "How ya doing?"

I didn't know how to respond or even if I should. So I just said, "I'm not unwell."

"That's the spirit!"

Then somebody else less cheery introduced himself as the anesthesiologist and said this won't hurt a bit, and the next thing I knew, the surgery was over and it apparently had gone well. That's how the stuff works. One minute you are telling yourself it will never work and the next thing you know you are unconscious; but you don't know it, if you know what I mean.

I was groggy as hell when I woke up, and I really did not know what was going on. I could see, but it was a few seconds before I could speak and that's a scary feeling. I saw a bunch of people in those green doctor outfits standing by a sink or two and cleaning things that appeared to be tools, and I blurted out, "What the hell is going on!" One of the nurses glanced over at me and said, "You're coming out of the anesthesia," with the unmistakable tone of "Men, they're such babies" in her voice.

The next thing I knew it was night, and I was in another strange place called intensive care. It was kind of frightening, just the fact that I was here and what I was here for, but there were plenty of nurses around, and now and then a doctor would stroll by, usually giving orders to someone.

For some reason they keep it kind of dark in intensive care, maybe to highlight the fright aspect. I had a little television that was about two inches from my head on the left side, so I just watched movies until I fell asleep, which is the best thing to do when there isn't much else to do.

The next day I was in a regular hospital room with a window and lights and a phone; and just outside the door was a reception area, and there were lots of people everywhere. I felt much better and safer. It was sunny outside and the future looked bright. I have no recollection of having been moved from intensive care to the other room. One of the nurses told me the anesthesia has residual effects for a few hours, and that's why I don't remember. Funny I can recall some things, but not others. Oh well.

Anyway, that morning, a doctor I'd never seen before stepped into the room and tossed a couple of bottles of pills on my bed and said, "You gotta take these. You gotta." And then he left.

While I was in the hospital, everybody from Dr. C's office came to see me. They were all worried about me with the surgery, and Dr. C told me I was the subject of all the conversations in her office, which made me feel like a celebrity, except that I was in a hospital bed with gauze in my nose and a catheter. The gauze was there because the surgeon goes into the brain through the nose and pushes aside anything that is in the way and—ah, never mind. You get the idea.

After three days of watching *Gilligan's Island* on television, I was sent home. I got a taxi.

The surgeon said the surgery went fine, and so did the doctor who had tossed me the pills, which were to keep my thyroid up and my blood pressure down. I had every reason to believe I was OK now, so I went back to work after two weeks, and everyone at least pretended to be glad to see me. It's funny, when you tell people you had brain surgery, they always look at your head with curiosity, maybe to see if there's still room for a brain.

It was good to be back to normal and have all that behind me. And two weeks later the surgeon called and said they had to go in again.

I had to go in for another round of surgery. Apparently once was not enough. Did they not take it seriously the first time? This was brain surgery, after all. I would think they wouldn't want to goof around, but I don't know. I'm not a doctor. Heck, I don't even play one on TV.

The conversation with the surgeon-boy went like this:

Me: Why do I need more surgery?

Him: Because we didn't get all the tumor out.

Me: Why not?

Him: Because it was too close to the optic nerve.

Me: Well, isn't it still too close to the optic nerve?

Him: Yes, but we're going to be more aggressive this time.

Me: This was just two weeks ago. Couldn't you have been aggressive then?

Him: Yes, but it was too close to the optic nerve . . .

Okay, so I have to say I did not understand anything about surgery, brain tumors, or anything else regarding this Acromegaly deal, but this sounded odd to me. I talked with Dr. C about it, and she agreed. She set me up with a different surgeon, a fellow who is world famous in this field; and his name also starts with C, so let's call him Dr. C Note.

Dr. C Note was more like it, an older guy with plenty of experience and a calm and friendly manner. And he looked like Barry Morse, the actor who played Gerard on *The Fugitive*, so he was cool with me.

The surgeon calling me about the second surgery called around Christmas. I told him I would have to think about it. I would eventually agree to it, and surgery with Dr. C Note was in April of the following year. That gave me lots of time to worry about my health and future. Here I had a brain tumor, not a cold or a virus, or even pneumonia. A tumor, in my brain. What the hell?

Living my somewhat normal life was very strange over the last several months. One day I didn't even know I was ill, and the next day I find out about a tumor in my—what? hand? foot?—no, my *brain*.

One morning I was seated at a table at my favorite local coffee shop, which was packed to the walls with other customers. Still, the sounds of clanging silverware and the various machines did not break me from my reverie. I had been thinking about my mom, who passed away the December before I was first diagnosed, and how I had wanted to sneak back home for the holidays and surprise her. But I couldn't, because she was suddenly gone. I started crying and I didn't want to, not in a public place, but I couldn't help it.

I put down my coffee cup and turned toward the wall. A little girl was standing with her mother as she waited for her order, and the girl asked her why that man was crying. Her mother said she didn't know. The little girl walked over to me and looked at me.

"Hey, mister," she said, "don't cwy." Then she patted my head with a little hand. And that, naturally, made me cry even more.

The second surgery went much better, not that I'd know from experience; I was unconscious the whole time. But more doctors talked with me afterwards and told me they took more of the tumor out, but not all of it because it was dangerously close to the carotid artery, which is not something you want to fool around with. A good portion of the pituitary came out with it, which meant I would need medication.

Since Dr. C had set me up with the folks at Northwestern Medical, down in the Loop area of the big, bad city, I was going there more often. I was under the care of an endocrine doctor with a different initial, Doctor M, and he got me taking an injection that provides for the body what the pituitary would, were it still in place and all there. I took it once every six months, the main problem being that I still had (and have) growth hormone issues.

I didn't notice any difference while taking this medication, but it seemed to be working. Thanks to insurance, it cost $35 a month, which I'd rather not have to pay, but what the hell? If it kept me alive a little longer, how bad could it be?

After a year or so, I started getting billed three grand per month, which I definitely didn't want to pay, and I just kind of drifted away from the whole thing—the doctors, the medication.

Just after the surgery is when I met Sal, my aforementioned girlfriend. We first saw each other in the same coffee shop, The Metropolis Café on Chicago's North Side. One night I was practicing my card trick routines, and Sal had been sitting on a couch near the front door. She came over and sat across from me at my table and said, "Alright, show me something."

I assumed she meant magic, so that's what I did. I had seen her around the place a few times as she talked with other people, and I liked her long blonde hair and how, as she spoke, she had sort of a crooked smile, which made her look even more beautiful.

She was a school teacher (still is, in fact) who taught algebra to eighth graders. She thought it was cool that I worked at a bookstore and was a semi professional magician. We both learned a lot about each other that very first night, and I eventually met her roommate and best friend, Jenny; happily, they lived just a few blocks away from me.

As the months went by I could not bring myself to tell Sal about my Acromegaly. I don't know why, really. It was a hard secret to keep, especially since we spent so much time together.

One thing is for sure: after not taking any medication for a couple of years, my mind was getting plenty foggy. I didn't know if it showed at work or with Sal until I had taken to losing my balance and falling down, usually outside. So I figured it would be a good time to let Sal know about all this.

I told her one evening when we stopped by the Metropolis before going home, and her reactions were not what I had expected.

“Why the fuck did you stop taking the injections?” she asked, sitting across from me at our usual table.

“Because it was too expensive.”

“But your company straightened it all out. What the hell?”

When I initially filled her in on the surgeries and all, she just sat quietly and wide eyed, her mouth forming an O and a million questions developing across her face.

One night I was walking home from the library, and I got dizzy and fell on the sidewalk and busted my head up pretty good, blood pouring into my eyes and a headache on its way. I was just two blocks from home so I walked to my building. Sal was standing on the sidewalk out front, and when she saw me she looked terrified. She also wanted to know if I had forgotten we were taking Jenny out for drinks for her birthday.

She cleaned me up in my bathroom and told me I should stay home and Jenny would understand. It’s nice to have someone care about you.

But I blew it. I always blow it, but I didn’t want to blow it this time. But I did.

One night we were watching television, and Sal was telling me about stuff at work. I have to say I was having trouble following what she was saying, and it showed.

She moved her face right up into mine and shouted, “Where are you?!”

She said I’d been too distant for too long, and she took that to mean that I didn’t like her anymore, and I almost started crying (I’m a crybaby, so what?) when she said, “That’s it,” and she got her purse and left.

I looked out the window and saw her crossing the street ten stories below. I always liked watching her walk because of this cute knock-kneed way she had about her, but this time she was walking away, and I thought about what I’d done wrong because I do everything wrong, from childhood on up, with people yelling at me all the time, like my dad, who always said I would never amount to anything, and I stood watching Sal walk away because this time she was not walking away to go home or to go to work, this time she was walking away from me, and I still get tears in my eyes every time I think about that night.

One day I got a letter in the mail from Doctor M, and he invited me to be part of a study for a new medication that was similar to what I was already on. I decided to take him up on that because I needed to get back to being healthy again. I was too groggy all the time, and my legs and shoulders hurt all day. And I was not doing well at work. After Sal left I didn't do much of anything but watch TV, and I wanted to change this lifestyle. I was also becoming scared all the time again, thinking I was going to fall and do serious damage or I was going to have a stroke or heart attack or both, or monsters were going to get me or something would go wrong.

Doctor M introduced me to a research endocrine nurse named Daphne, and she would guide me through this study of the new medication. For a while it seemed the same, but the injection was once a month and would control my insulin-like growth factor levels, something I did not know I had, until I learned it was growth hormone related. Daphne taught me how to do this injection on my own. I could do it at home all by myself. It wasn't easy to learn, at least not for me. You stab yourself with a giant needle and plunge it on in, but it goes slow because the medication is really thick. When she does the injection, I don't feel anything, and she taught me how to do it the same way. She also took the time to contact a company that offers patients financial support, and it eventually cost me nothing. Just my style!

Daphne is quite remarkable. She actually has an honest interest in my health and cares what happens, and she stays on top of things to make sure I take the medication.

She also got me involved with the company that markets the medication, and they send me around to various cities to talk about my diagnosis and whatever else comes to mind.

Who knew being sick could actually be fun?

I soon started feeling normal again—no pain in my arms or legs, I can move around much better, and I don't fall down on a regular basis anymore. And that fogginess in my mind has cleared up (for the most part). At work I'm in charge of the multimedia department, and on Tuesdays I put out the new releases, an activity that used to take me a week to complete. But now it only takes a couple of hours.

After the second surgery I had a round of Gamma Knife radiation, and that was one day I have no fond memories of. You sit alone for hours with a metal helmet screwed into your head, you are escorted into a dark room much like the MRI place, and you lie down while the doctor and his assistant shoot laser beams at you, but not before running back to a soundproof booth. Talk about scary. I had to lie there by myself while they talked in the booth. Since it was soundproofed, I only assume they were talking, and I didn't really completely understand what was going on. As you probably guessed, I started crying as I was waiting for this procedure to end. This whole thing has been frightening from the start, and I've always heard that radiation can do all kinds of thing to you, like generate cancer. I don't know if that's true, but it got me to worrying plenty. But after it was finally over, I spent the night in the hospital upstairs, and I got to watch television and eat ice cream, so it wasn't all bad.

But I'm not worried anymore. I still have Acromegaly and I probably always will, but I'm in good hands now—with Daphne and Dr. C on my side, I feel plenty safe.

I saw Sal recently while I was visiting the Metropolis, where I had not been in a couple of years because I had moved out of that neighborhood. She explained that she was afraid that the real me was fading away because of my lack of interest in my health, and she wanted the old me back, and that's why she left, and I can certainly understand. There's worse reason for someone to say goodbye.

My feelings on death have changed for the better, I think. I no longer worry about it. If it happens, it happens. Can't do much about it afterwards. I'd prefer not to have this illness, but since I do, it makes for something interesting to talk about wherever you go.

Michael Cookman is a multimedia coordinator with Borders Books and Music and a part-time professional magician living in Evanston, Illinois. He has performed magic for John Denver, Gloria Estefan, and Sonny Bono, just to drop a few names. Michael was diagnosed with Acromegaly in 2002 and has written about the illness on various blogs (Salon.com for one) and has spoken publicly about Acromegaly for Consensus Medical and the Ipsen Company. Michael proudly serves on the inaugural Board of Directors for Acromegaly Community.

Life around Surgery

Michael Carroll

All human situations have their inconveniences. We feel those of the present but neither see nor feel those of the future; and hence we often make troublesome changes without amendment, and frequently for the worse.

—Benjamin Franklin

Two thousand eight was an interesting year for me and for my family. My mother uses the word *interesting* to describe my birth, which happened 30 years earlier . . . maybe it was because I was over twelve pounds. Two thousand eight was the year I was introduced to the word *Acromegaly* and everything that went with it. I've learned that everyone's journey to the diagnosis is unique, and my experience only confirms this belief. In 2008 I had a pregnant wife, a young daughter, a job with a company that was in jeopardy, and two major surgeries. I also learned three key lessons: 1) football can save your life, 2) not every bad thing that happens to you is actually a bad thing, and 3) the many faces of fear. First, though, a walk down memory lane . . .

In 1994 I was the last child left in the house. My sister was married, and both of my brothers already had jobs and homes of their own. My parents had planned well, enabling them to retire to Florida in their fifties. Coming from New York, I thought the post-retirement move to Florida was actually state law.

I started playing football when I was nine, following in the footsteps of both of my brothers, and my dad was my first coach. While I *hated* football in the beginning, ultimately I grew to love the game. I think it was my love of football that made me excited for the move. After all, football in Florida is the stuff of legend to a teenage boy, and I looked forward to being a part of it. While being the new kid in any school can be very difficult, being on the football team is a fantastic ice breaker. I quickly worked my way into the starting lineup as a starting guard (no one pulled around the corner and blocked downfield better than I did). Even better, the team got off to a great start.

Our school was ranked in the Top 5 for schools of our size in Florida, which is a tremendous accomplishment, and everyone took practice pretty seriously because of this. One warm (is there any other kind in Florida?) Wednesday afternoon during practice, I was filling in at running back for the practice squad offense against the starting defense. The day was proceeding as any other, with the practice squad performing well and even scoring a couple of times. And then it happened. I took the ball on a handoff, planning to dive to the right side. Unfortunately there was no hole for me to run through, and I was not a dynamic enough runner to move much more than straight ahead. Defenders had each of my legs, and out of the corner of my eye, I saw a shadow that looked like night was falling; but unfortunately for me, it was our 280-pound defensive tackle. When his head connected with mine, night did fall, at least temporarily! I woke up a few moments after hitting the ground and tried to get up, but my legs wouldn't cooperate. I made it a few feet before collapsing. As everyone gathered around me, I remember asking a question—"Ice cream?" I thought someone had offered me ice cream and was actually somewhat annoyed that no one had any. While I had suffered a serious neck injury, I did the football player move: after a few minutes I got up and "walked it off." The trainer decided that I had nothing more serious than a "stinger," which is a nice name for a spinal cord shock. My parents met with the coach that day, and he told them that I had been shaken up, but no one took it very seriously.

The next morning I woke up and tried to get ready for school, but I had a horrible burning sensation up and down my arms and legs. To call it *pins and needles* would be overly charitable; *pins and napalm* might have worked better. It was the remnants of the neurological trauma I had sustained the day before. I told Mom and Dad about it, and they quickly scheduled an appointment with their neurologist. The appointment wasn't until the afternoon, which was fine with me because that day was an important day for a Catholic School boy: Ring Ceremony. This meant three important things to me: 1) no uniforms, 2) shortened classes, and 3) I would receive my dad's high school ring because mine hadn't arrived yet. I was very excited and didn't want to miss the day. Unfortunately, sometimes fate has a sense of humor; and as I drove to school, my car broke down. So there I was, weakened, uncomfortable, late, and pushing a 1986 Plymouth Duster hatchback down the street to a gas station. Thankfully some classmates saw me and gave me a ride to school.

The day proceeded quickly, and after the ring ceremony Mom and Dad took me to the doctor. Little did I know at the time that it was to be the first of what would be many trips to neurologists and neurosurgeons in my lifetime. Dr. Sunter listened carefully to what had happened and immediately ordered an MRI of my cervical spine. Unfortunately MRIs are not like x-rays; you don't get immediate results. The two weeks I had to wait seemed a lot longer. When we finally got the phone call, the receptionist hinted that something did not look good in the MRI, and my parents tried to prepare me by dropping hints like, "What will you do if you can't play football anymore?" I'd mumble something about focusing on my studies or getting into other activities. I didn't catch on because the idea that I wouldn't be able to play football anymore was unfathomable.

When the day came to hear the MRI results, I was so nervous that I was twitching while I waited. Dr. Sunter walked in and told us that the results were in. He turned on the light board with the results on it and then quickly turned it back off. "Let's go look at a model of a normal spinal column." He pulled out a model, showing me all of the other important components of a healthy spinal column, checking for my understanding.

"Good," he said. "Now let's go look at yours."

"That can't be good," I thought.

We walked back to the board, and he turned the light back on. I immediately noticed a problem, now that I knew what a healthy spinal column looked like. Dr. Sunter explained that I had herniated three discs in my neck. "I'll have to thank Terrence (the boy that laid the hit on me)," I sarcastically thought.

The team moved on without me, but I was still involved as a kind of unofficial assistant to the coach, handling offensive duties, especially the offensive line. Coach Bernie, as we called him, really helped pull me through the darkest of those days. I still have a card that he gave me right after I had gotten the bad news. It was a get well soon card, but on the inside flap, Coach Bernie wrote to me, in his own words, about how proud he was of me and the strength I had shown through my ordeal. I used my experience to write a heck of a college essay. They asked me about a time when I was forced to adapt to changing circumstances in life. Boy, did I hit that one out of the park! I went from football to acting in the Drama Club; I got great grades, began teaching Sunday School, worked part time, and had a number of other activities. I guess my ability to adapt to stressful situations would prove to be a tremendous asset when I was later diagnosed with Acromegaly.

I know I've spent a lot of time on a football injury that happened in high school. This is a book about Acromegaly after all! The thing about an Acromegaly diagnosis, though, is that it is incredibly difficult to come by. Acromegaly is insidious, presenting with a variety of seemingly unrelated symptoms. Often the diagnosis comes after the disease has done a large amount of damage. I was blessed because I was diagnosed early, at age thirty, and this happened entirely because of the neck injury I had suffered fourteen years earlier.

* * *

On Christmas Eve, 2007 I was living in Las Vegas. I was married and had a two-year-old little girl named Madeline. Theresa, my wife, was pregnant with our second child. Mom and Dad were staying at our house for the holidays because Mom and Dad are incredible and always make the effort to be with us. Dad and I decided to go golfing on Christmas Eve. I picked the game up after the football injury, and I love golfing with my dad. That evening we enjoyed a traditional Christmas Eve dinner, and it warmed my heart to watch my wife, daughter, and mom all working together in the kitchen. After Madeline went to bed, Theresa and I went to work on the best part of Christmas: being my daughter's Santa Claus. First I ate a couple of the cookies that Madeline had set out, and Theresa ate some of the carrots (she's thin, and a vegetarian). Mom and Dad sat on the couch as we slowly filled the living room with presents. By the time we were done, there was no visible floor in the room, and my parents were staring at us as if we were both quite insane. We were both very excited that this was the first Christmas when Madeline would understand what was happening, and having another baby on the way only made it more special.

I awoke earlier than everyone, at 4:00 a.m. I'm not normally an early riser, but the excruciating pain in my right hand made it very difficult to keep sleeping. I didn't wake anyone; I just continued to lie on the couch wondering when the pain would go away. I was used to waking up at night and finding my hands numb; usually if I shook them out, the numbness went away. This was something that had been going on for years. But the feeling that day was different. The numbness was there, but the pain was new, and when day finally broke I noticed that my right hand was swollen as well. Being a typical man, I popped some ibuprofen and went on with my day. I did tell Theresa about it but didn't make a big deal of it because I figured it would go away in no time, the way the numbness always did. In the back of my head, though, I knew that the neck injury was going to catch up with me eventually, and I figured that that may have been what was happening. But I did not want to dwell on that on Christmas Day.

On December 26 the pain hadn't gotten any better, and the hand was still swollen. We all thought that the football injury was coming back to cause problems, and Theresa and Mom said that everyone agreed that I should go to see the doctor. I went to see my regular doctor, and I told him about my neck injury from so many years ago. He prescribed a wrist splint, an anti-inflammatory, and a medication that should reduce the neurological symptoms, thinking it was related to carpal tunnel syndrome. Our plan was to try this for ten days, get through the holidays, and adjust if necessary.

The holidays came and went, Mom and Dad went home, and while the discomfort was improved, it was still a problem. Back to the doctor I went. He's a perceptive man, and he could tell that I was starting to become concerned that my problem was deeper than carpal tunnel. He called the neurologist while still in the exam room with me. The neurologist prescribed a steroid for the inflammation and told my doctor that his office would call to schedule me for an appointment. As I was getting up to leave, he rubbed my shoulders. I think he could sense my concern. He said, "Don't worry, we're going to get you fixed up."

I left the office and went right to the pharmacy to fill my prescription. After dropping off the slip, I strolled around the store waiting for my prescription. I flipped through the DVDs in the $5 bin and wondered what was really wrong with me. I did not believe that carpal tunnel was my problem. I grabbed an animated movie, *The Reef* I think, for Madeline and made my way back to the pharmacy.

The first day that I took this medication was a lot like taking an IV consisting of five gallons of energy drink. By eight thirty in the morning, I was at the park with Madeline. I climbed everything she climbed, went under everything she crawled through, pushed her on the swings, and chased her around. Afterwards we went to the convenience store to get some treats—we both love Slushies. We made it home around lunch time, and I started cleaning the house. By two in the afternoon, I had cleaned the house top to bottom, vacuumed, and cleaned the toilets. As Madeline took her nap, I went to the gym. When I came home I suggested that we go out to dinner somewhere. Theresa looked at me like I had gone crazy. She asked if I was going to stop moving at any point, and the way the steroid was coursing through my veins, I wasn't sure. I also wasn't sure if I would be able to fall asleep that night.

Thankfully, with each successive day of taking the steroid, the hyperactivity decreased. By the end of the next week, I had my first appointment with the neurologist. He was kind and thoughtful, and he had a rather thick accent, as I would expect from my other doctor's referral. He took a look at me and gave me the usual neurological exam that I had been through so many times as an athlete. He then prescribed an MRI and a nerve conductivity test and another course of steroids for me, which meant that I was going to be *very* active for at least another six days.

It was around this time that Theresa's all-day morning sickness kicked in. With Amelia (baby #2), Theresa was even sicker than with Madeline. Theresa was struggling and didn't have the energy to chase Madeline around, so I asked Mom to come for a few weeks. As always, Mom was eager to help, and she hopped on a plane the next day. She was just in time, too. As soon as she got to town, Theresa had a nasty reaction to one of the anti-nausea medications, which would actually lead to a visit to the hospital for a few days.

The ER was busy, so we were stuck in a chair in the hallway. As the hours passed, the first nurse, the only one who seemed to care about Theresa, took off. The doctors in ERs are overworked, so I didn't expect much from them, but the nurse that took over seemed to be less than thrilled with her career choice. At one point she and I had a strongly worded disagreement about the fact that we were there for the *doctor's* medical judgment, not hers. I felt that my wife's breathing would benefit from a bed and observation; she disagreed. Theresa's OB shared my opinion, so I guess I won. It didn't feel like winning, though, as I looked at Theresa holding a towel to her mouth to catch the saliva that was pouring out of her swollen lips, unable to take its normal course down her throat. At midnight Theresa wished me a happy birthday. It was the big 3-0 for me, and it was off to a hell of a start!

Theresa was finally discharged early in the evening on my birthday. We got in the car and drove home. When we walked through the door, I was confronted with black balloons and dead flowers. Mom had gone all out in celebration of my birthday. She and Theresa had been planning this for a few days: it's something of a family tradition that I started by sending my brother a funeral arrangement at his office on his thirtieth birthday. We all had the first laugh in a long time. Over the next few days, Theresa started feeling better and stronger, so Mom headed home.

The Saturday after Mom left, we all went back to my neurologist's office for the nerve conductivity test. This seems to be a test that was developed solely with the idea of torturing the prospective carpal tunnel patient. Between the bolts of electricity that are sent shooting down the nerves in your arms and the needles that are stuck into your muscle, there really isn't a lot to enjoy. The goal is to test the speed of your nerves. If you have carpal tunnel syndrome, it will take longer for the signal to reach the end of the line. The truth was, I was rooting for carpal tunnel because the alternative was a problem from my neck injury, and I was pretty sure that would lead to surgery.

I also went to get my MRI, as instructed. It had been a while since I had visited my dear old friend, the magnetic resonance imaging machine, and things had surely changed! Now they had a cage that they put your head in. That wasn't around in 1994. Also, they gave me headphones and tuned in to satellite radio for me—again, a luxury that wasn't around way-back-when. You've got to enjoy the little things, right? MRIs are a blast, as long as you aren't claustrophobic. Thankfully, I'm not. I barely fit into the machine, as I'm pretty broad shouldered. My nose *almost* brushes the top of the machine, as I also have a pretty huge head and a nose that a family of four could hide out under to escape the rain. Actually, it seemed as if my nose had been increasing in size, something I hadn't thought much about but which would become important later. After thirty minutes of the worst drum solo ever, I was slid out and sent on my way.

One thing I had forgotten after my initial injury is that the waiting is almost as bad as the injury itself. It is always *interminable.* In this case, it's not like I expected my neck to be better—far from it. My fear was, how much worse would it be? I had images of discs in my neck, exploded like jellyfish that had had M-80 firecrackers dropped on them. I imagined that every disc was going to have to be fused and that I wouldn't be able to turn my head, forever only seeing what was directly in front of me. No longer able to drive or even to look up. The mind can do horrible things to you when left unchecked. On top of that, rumblings had started at work that we (the company) were in serious financial trouble. The timing was perfect. I was facing an uncertain future with my neck, my wife was pregnant with our second child, and we were living 2,500 miles away from the closest family members.

At the end of February, I went back to see my neurologist for my diagnosis. I don't remember why, but Theresa and Madeline didn't come with me. Usually they do—they're my entourage, a couple of good-looking girls that I like to travel with. I look better just by being around them. The neurologist had yet to view the films, so when he joined me in the exam room and turned on the light board, we did not have a moment like the one with Dr. Sunter. Instead, he put the films on the board, looked, and quickly said, "Oh wow. Oh no. Oh sheet." Remember I mentioned that he had an accent? He was not talking about bedding. The worst disc was worse, and now the neighboring disc was showing signs of deterioration as well. He then told me that he was going to refer me to the neurosurgeon that he liked to work with, Dr. Gary Flangas.

I took the films with me and left, thinking, "It can't get much worse than this." I figured that my nightmare was going to come true. Four discs. All were going to have to be fused, and I would spend the next fifty years of my life walking around like a robot. Like I said, your mind can do horrible things. I went home and immediately started googling (doctors must hate the Internet, no?) words like *stenosis* and *anterior cervical discectomy with fusion*. Just your usual light reading. Theresa looked at me and accused me of going to the worst-case scenario. I looked back and explained that based upon what I had seen, I was the worst-case scenario. (Turns out I was wrong about that, and a little melodramatic.) Then I sat on the bed and started sobbing. I'm really not much of a crier, typically. I had noticed that since becoming a parent, I was more emotional. I mean, hearing Israel Kamakawiwo'ole sing "Somewhere Over the Rainbow" always got me misty eyed, as did the other usual things for men: Mufasa dying in *The Lion King*, Rudy Ruettiger getting carried off the field at the end of *Rudy*, and, of course, the entire end of *Red Dawn*. But when Madeline was born, I cried when I held her for the first time, and ever since, the most innocuous things bring tears to my eyes. This was different though; I was scared and overwhelmed. However, throughout my life, whenever I receive bad news, I am usually down in the dumps for the rest of the day; but when I wake up the next morning, I jump out of bed ready to kick the ass of whatever problem is in front of me.

I awoke rested and ready, true to form. I'm an optimist by nature, and I tend to believe that things work out for the best. I'm not an "Everything happens for a reason" person; there's a little too much predestination in that for me. But it was time to plan. First I called the neurosurgeon for an appointment; and then I called the radiologist for copies of the scan, and I charmed some extra copies out of him. I called Mom and asked her to reach out to her network—and her network was *vast.* I had no problem with seeing Dr. Flangas, but I didn't want to wait a month to get some answers. Again, the waiting. I would handle it as best I could, but if I could shorten the wait, I would.

Ultimately, I saw a neurosurgeon who seemed disinterested. I was also due to go out of town on business for ten days. Prior to my trip, I needed some new pants and a pair of shoes. I hadn't bought shoes in a while and was surprised that my shoe size had gone from a 10½ to a 13. "That's weird," I told Madeline. She was two, so she didn't know what I was talking about. She was busy walking around in size 12 hiking boots anyway. I didn't think about the shoe thing again, until three weeks later.

My trip passed both quickly and slowly, and when I got back it was time to see Dr. Flangas. I was scheduled for the afternoon, so I went to work first. Then I went home before the appointment and picked up Theresa and Madeline. Like I said, we stick together on these things. We were called into the exam room. It had a nice view of the parking lot and the highway. I was looking for any way that I could think of to distract myself. Theresa was keeping Madeline busy. Madeline had spent a lot of time in doctors' offices over the last few months and had really become a very well behaved little girl.

Dr. Flangas came in after probably twenty minutes, though it seemed longer than that. We introduced ourselves, and I immediately began calling him "Doc." I call all of my doctors "Doc," and I have no idea why. We started talking about my neck. I went through the whole background: football injury when young, numbness fourteen years later, concerned, carpal tunnel, steroids . . . blah, blah, blah.

He looked at me and said, "I think you have carpal tunnel."

I said, "But my neck . . ."

He said, "Well, I think you have carpal tunnel caused by Acromegaly."

I responded with, "You just made up a word." Seriously, *Acromegaly*? What, were we playing Mad-Libs or something? I can be very mature sometimes.

Dr. Flangas explained Acromegaly in the simplest of terms. He told me that it is typically caused by a growth hormone–secreting tumor on the pituitary gland. My blank stare must have concerned him, but he sounded a lot like Charlie Brown's teacher, only I could make out some of his words, like *tumor*, *head*, *brain*. I could imagine him reaching deep into his reserve of patience to explain it to me. He asked me if I knew who André the Giant was. I answered in the affirmative. He explained that André had this type of tumor, but developed it as a child, which caused his gigantism. If I had it, I had developed it after I had stopped growing, which only caused really, and I mean *really*, weird shit to happen to the body.

I decided to bring the conversation back to any area that I was more comfortable with, in this case, my neck. I said, "Will fixing my neck get rid of my headaches?"

He looked at me and with exasperation said, "Your neck, your neck. We'll fix your neck. Tell me more about your headaches."

I had been having these headaches for years. I first became aware of them back in 2004, when we were still living in Los Angeles. I called them Tsunami Headaches. I could feel the headache coming on, slowly rolling over my head. Then it would crest and crash. I would be completely debilitated for a few minutes. Then it would slowly recede and be gone. If I was driving when I felt one coming on, I had to pull over. They were painful enough to bring tears to my eyes; few things ever hurt me more. Dr. Flangas listened carefully, and it was clear that he didn't think these headaches were caused by my neck injury.

He asked Theresa if I looked different than when we first met. She said that I did. My nose was bigger, and there were other subtle changes. Then a light bulb went off for me. I mentioned the increased shoe size. He nodded. Then I remembered something that had bothered me for a while. I had developed an underbite over the two years preceding this appointment. I used to have perfectly aligned teeth as a result of braces I had had when I was eight years old (my teeth had been *really* crooked). I had noticed now that my lower teeth protruded past my upper teeth. When I asked my dentist about it, he just tried to push my jaw back into place. He wasn't a great dentist.

Sitting there, it made sense. It explained so much. But the downside was, it meant I had a tumor in my head. At least it wasn't cancerous. I again tried to explain everything through the neck injury, and Dr. Flangas simply said, "It's carpal tunnel. I'm ordering a pituitary MRI, and we'll see you back here in a few weeks."

I walked out in a stupor. All I kept thinking was "braintumorbraintumorbraintumor." It was on an unending loop in my cruel mind. I didn't even know yet if I had tumor or not, but that was all I could think about. As we were driving home, I was quiet. I had gone in thinking I was going to have neck surgery, and I was, but this had completely blindsided me. I told Theresa that I couldn't believe this! A tumor! She said (again), "You always go to the worst case." I just looked at her, caught somewhere between confusion and disbelief. It's actually the same look I would have given the dog if one day she said, "You know, this dog food isn't very good. I like cat food." Seriously, it was that surprising to me. I think I said, "Ooooookaaaaay." We went home, and I consulted Google, MD (again).

What I learned was pretty startling. One thing, Acromegaly is extremely rare. Secondly, it is not easy to find websites explaining it. Many websites had copies of an article from a doctor in Boston, just reprinted. Then I came across a website that listed the symptoms pretty comprehensively. I'll address these in bullet-point format—they are that interesting:

- Soft tissue swelling of the hands and feet – Yup, I had that.
- Change in ring and shoe size – Had that too. Discovered during the shoe shopping trip with Madeline.
- Bony changes that alter the facial features – Batting 1.000 so far. My jaw was and is much larger.

- Overgrowth of bone and cartilage leading to arthritis – I had been battling knee pain for a few years and even had arthroscopic surgery on my right knee a year and a half before the word *Acromegaly* entered my life. Count it, as they say in basketball.
- Thick, coarse, oily skin – Uh-huh.
- Skin tags – This is getting ridiculous, I thought. Yup.
- Enlarged lips, nose, and tongue – My nose, while never small, was definitely bigger, as was my tongue. Sometimes it felt like my tongue didn't fit right in my mouth. And my nose had been the source of many family jokes over the past few years. An example, and one of my favorites, came from my brother. He said that of course my neck needed surgery; it had been holding my nose up for years. Of course, I told him that if I did have a tumor that caused my nose growth he would have to apologize. I win! I guess . . . not really.
- Deepening of the voice due to enlarged sinuses and vocal cords – I was all over this one. I already had a deep voice, but it had definitely gotten quite a bit deeper according to Theresa. A theme seemed to be developing.
- Excessive sweating and skin odor – Sadly, yes. In fact, one day the boss called me into his office to tell me that I had smelled incredibly bad the day before. At that moment I knew he was a true friend, and a bit of a dick (kidding!). Theresa had also been recommending for years that I should reapply deodorant through the course of the day.
- Fatigue and weakness – Maybe yes, maybe no. Hard to tell when you have a toddler. Call it a push.
- Headaches – Oh yeah.
- Impaired vision – I have had corrective lenses for a long time, so probably unrelated. Our first no!
- Reduced sex drive – In some ways I was as bothered by the body odor thing, to be honest, but this one was still a yes. At least there might be an explanation.

That's a great big list, and pretty diverse, but not comprehensive. The symptoms for Acromegaly are pretty diverse as well. My final tally against this score card was 11 yeses, 1 push, and 1 no. According to Dr. Google, there was no way I didn't have Acromegaly.

The next day I scheduled my pituitary MRI. I also told my boss/friend Mark about what was happening. He told me not to worry, that he was sure things would work out. I always wonder when people say things like that; how the hell do they know? After all, all I could think about was my daughter, the baby on the way, and the possible tumor in my head. Still, when Mark said it, I did find comfort in his words; he has a way about him on these things. But here we were, back to the waiting game. I also told Mom and Dad what was going on, and I asked them not to tell anyone else. We don't like to get people needlessly worried, and my siblings have their own lives and troubles, like anyone else. There would be a time to talk to them about things, but not yet.

Stress can manifest itself in strange ways, and there is no stress quite like unknown medical problems. One day, as I was sitting with a colleague, the president of the company walked into the office and closed the door. He proceeded to berate us about returning sales calls, saying he had heard that we weren't calling people back. He had been particularly rough on me because he viewed me as loyal to the CEO and not to him. I was angered by his comments because it was only through the efforts of my colleague Mark and me that any business was coming in to the company. I then said, "You know the benefit of the doubt would be nice." The president then launched into an expletive-laden tirade.

I responded, "Shouting obscenities, questioning our work ethic and impugning our integrity is your idea of respectful speech?"

He turned beet red and started screaming at me, finishing with, "I've never spoken to you with anything but respect, so shut the HELL up."

I launched out of my chair, prepared to put him through the wall. This was going to be no easy feat as he had two inches and one hundred pounds on me, but I was pretty fit at the time. I told him that if he ever said anything else it would be the last thing he said until they unwired his jaw. Thankfully someone broke us up before

I got to him. Ironically, he and our CEO would get into a fistfight a few months later, leading to both of them getting terminated from the company. But not before wreaking some more havoc on my life. By rights I should have been fired on the spot. I was completely insubordinate. Mark told me later that I did the right thing, because no one should speak to anyone as disrespectfully as our boss spoke to us.

I was definitely losing my composure; the stress was getting to me, the fear was getting to me, and the unknown was making it even worse. I went and got the MRI. It was actually two MRIs, one of the brain and one of the pituitary. The pituitary MRI took longer because the machine needed its sensitivity increased for an accurate image. I couldn't help but feel the pressure of the technician's gaze as I walked out. It seemed like he was looking at me, wondering what could be so wrong that I needed those scans taken.

Time actually sped up a little at this point. Mom came for a visit now that Theresa was feeling better. It was nice to have her in town. The visit was needed. I called the doctor's office every day to see if the results had been sent. My follow-up appointment was for the day after Mom left. We tried not to talk too much in front of Theresa, but whenever we had time to ourselves, Mom and I discussed what I should do if it turned out that I did have Acromegaly. On the Friday before my appointment, the office said that the scans had come back. I asked them to send me a copy to read, and they agreed. When I saw the fax come in, I couldn't read it fast enough. It said, "MRI of normal brain." I actually felt relieved and insulted at the same time! Normal brain? What was that supposed to mean??? Anyway, the report didn't say anything about a tumor, but it did mention "fullness in the area of the pituitary," which seemed weird. I was relieved though. No tumor it seemed. Theresa actually thought that this was bad news in a way. She thought that having the tumor stunk, but at least it explained all the weird things that were happening to my body. I saw her point, but I also thought that no tumor was good news.

Finally, it was Tuesday. I was on pins and needles all day despite what the report had said. We waited and waited and waited. It was actually only ten minutes, but it felt longer. Then Dr. Flangas walked through the door, and he did something that I truly appreciated and doctors never do: he got straight to the point. No foreplay, no disseminating. He said, "I was right. You do have a pituitary tumor." I remember my body's reaction very clearly. I felt my stomach drop, my tongue went dry, my vision contracted if that makes sense, and it felt like my eyes were shaking quickly from side to side. Mostly though, I remember the noise. I heard a rushing in my ears like a locomotive. I guess it was probably the blood coursing through my veins, but I never asked Dr. Google about it.

I could feel Theresa behind me, staring at my back. Madeline was gloriously oblivious. I squared my shoulders, lifted my head, found my voice, and said, "What's next?" My voice came out much stronger than I expected. Doc put the scans on the board and pointed at the little SOB that was causing all this weirdness in my body. He then explained what we would do to it but said that a total cure was very difficult to achieve. Then he said that we would fix the worst disc in my neck first because he had to get pretty aggressive with my neck for the Acromegaly surgery, so he wanted to have the neck strong first. That made sense to me, but I was still trying to not throw up. Then he called his assistant Natalie into the room. He told her that I appeared to have Acromegaly and that it was time to get my team together. I looked at her and said, "I win!" Typical man I guess, but I was trying to break the tension. Theresa gave me a dirty look.

I left the office in a daze. How the hell did this happen? I had a neck problem, that was all. Now I have a brain tumor, a pregnant wife, and an unsure work situation; and we live thousands of miles from family. As I floated down the hallway, Theresa touched my arm and said, "Are you okay?" Of course I wasn't . . . but I told her that I would be. Now we could make another plan. The uncertainty was gone.

I called Mom and Dad and told them the news. They kept a brave face on, but were deeply concerned. Mom decided to start calling everyone she knew in the medical community and all of the major medical centers in the country to see who was best at the procedure I would need done. I knew an issue was going to arise with Mom, but I didn't feel like dealing with it yet. One step at a time, as they say. Mom was going to want me to get the surgery done in New

York, or Boston, or wherever they specialize in pituitary tumors. I was pretty sure that I was going to want Dr. Flangas to do it. I felt very comfortable with him already. Not a fight I felt like having though. I also asked Mom to call my siblings; I was in no mood to hop on the phone with them.

Next I called Mark. I left him this message: "Hey, Mark, it's Junior." (Mark is MC, Sr. I am MC, Jr. We are not actually related.) "I just left the doctor, and the news wasn't good. I have a tumor the size of a grape on my pituitary. Give me a call when you have a chance." Mark called me back soon after and said, "Michael, listen, when they go in to remove this thing, make sure they take out the right grape-sized object. I would hate for them to remove your brain by accident." He and I laughed for five minutes after that; it was just what I needed. Total tension breaker for me. I discussed how I wanted to handle things at work. We were a small company, and I didn't want everyone to know about this. We agreed that I would tell a few critical senior managers the next day, and no one else. I did not want my life and dealings with other people to become about this. I didn't want anyone's sympathy, and I certainly didn't want anyone's pity. It's just not my style.

Theresa and I were pretty down the rest of the night. I think we picked up some Mexican food and went home. Mexican food is our comfort food; we love it to a point that is definitely unhealthy. We went to bed that night with some comfort—at least we knew what we were going to face, and now we could get to planning. I said it before, I love developing a strategy, and it was "get up and go" time!

The next morning I awoke and had that blissful thirty seconds between when I woke up and when I remembered what was happening in my life and to my body. When I went to sleep at night, I knew that I would have that moment in the morning when I would be temporarily ignorant. Theresa and I talked strategy. We felt the best thing to do was compartmentalize everything. First, the neck surgery and then Amelia's birth; finally, the brain surgery. While I know that it is in fact pituitary surgery, which is not technically the brain, my surgeon called it brain surgery, and I decided that since it was my head, I would call it whatever I wanted. Sadly, I had a friend debate the semantics of it with me; we aren't friends anymore.

I went to work, and Mark brought me in to his office. He sat me down and told me not to worry about anything. He told me that as long as he was part of the company, I would be taken care of. He made it clear to me how important I was to him and to the company and how much he cared about me and my family. It helped me put my mind somewhat at ease. I also told the president because I felt obligated, not because I wanted to. After all, I was only a few days removed from almost physically assaulting him.

Once back in the office, actually doing work was pretty much out of the question. Theresa had made it clear that she wanted to be my quarterback for everything. She wanted to keep my calendar, make my appointments, and keep track of prescriptions and everything else. She already had a filing system in place. The team was ready to go! I began researching—first the neck surgery, then the brain surgery. I checked with specialists to see if they took my insurance, just in case. Then I called my oldest friend, Holly, who was a nurse. We don't speak a lot, but we are still quite close. She asked how things were going, and I danced around it for a bit. Finally I got down to it and told her that I had Acromegaly. She refused to believe me. I was accused of googling rare conditions and playing a joke on her. To be fair, it is not out of the question that I would do something along those lines, but obviously I was telling the truth this time. She finally believed me and became concerned. I started asking her questions about the procedure because she had been a nurse for ten years at that point. She said that neither surgery was a picnic, but that I would get through them fine. Later, I found out that when she told her mother about my Acromegaly, her mother didn't believe it either! I guess I'm pretty good with my jokes!

The next few weeks were a whirlwind of appointments. The first was a stress test to make sure that I was healthy enough for surgery. After all of the tests, Jacques—my cardiologist and, ironically enough, a board member at the company—sat and talked with us for over an hour. We spent four hours total at his office that day. It was very funny; actually, he walked in, looked at me, and said, "Now I see it." Turns out I had a cardiologist who had also done a fellowship in endocrinology, as luck would have it. Despite feeling pretty low, things were actually working in my favor. I wouldn't call me lucky . . . and yet I would. I had stumbled in front of the right doctors, and I learned at this appointment that my condition was caught before any damage had been done to my heart. Jacques told me that I was healthy enough for my surgery.

I had a few things to take care of before the first surgery. First, I realized that Theresa and I needed a will. Theresa didn't want to talk about it, but we agreed that if anything happened to us, we would want Madeline and Amelia (not born yet) to go with my brother and his wife. I also looked into getting life insurance. When I had left my last job, I was irresponsible and didn't get a plan of my own. Theresa didn't want to have these conversations, but to me it was important.

We needed to do the math on how much the surgeries were going to cost. Thankfully, I had very good health insurance. I knew that I had an $8,000 out-of-pocket maximum, which we would have to come up with, but overall I wasn't terribly concerned. That is, until I learned from Mark that the president of the company wanted to lay me off rather than pay me during my recovery time. Mark told me that he would never let that happen, and I believed him, but WOW! What a slap. I had moved my family to work for this guy's company, left a good job, suffered through the dark days; and when I ran into tough times of my own, this asshole wanted to fire me! The company had been going through a round of layoffs, and senior managers were taking pay cuts. He figured that letting me go would mean he could keep his salary where it was. Mark made it clear that I was critical to the company's success and that I was not to be touched. It was funny: my friend who had brought me to the company did nothing at all, but Mark, who I'd only known for six months, was there to protect me and my family. It was a relief knowing that I would have a job as long as the company existed.

The weekend before the surgery, Mark and I went golfing. He was staying in town, and Theresa was spending time with her father as he received an award. I wanted to take advantage of my temporary bachelorhood. I don't like to go golfing when my girls are home. I can only go on the weekend, and you know that you aren't going to be home for at least eight hours. "Who knows?" I thought. "This might be the last time I go golfing." Not a healthy way to think, but realistic.

After the round we went back to my house where I had been marinating some rib-eye steaks for two days, and I thought that steak and beer were the perfect way to end the day. Mark hung out for a while, sensing my nervousness, I think. We decided to settle down by watching *300.* Nothing settles the nerves like a "swords and sandals" flick, I suppose. I didn't do much on Sunday. I played some *Madden* on the Wii. I knew I wasn't going to be able to do that for a while either. The day passed slowly as thoughts of my first surgery crossed my mind.

Mom flew in the next day, thankfully making it so that I was no longer alone. I still felt lonely though; it's hard to explain. Ever since the diagnosis, I had an inner monologue going. It had changed from "braintumorbraintumorbraintumor." Now I heard a constant scream in my head that went "IT'S IN THERE RIGHT NOW!!!!" Not a fun thing to keep hearing in your head, nonstop, every day since the diagnosis. Even if I was in the middle of a conversation with someone, I would still hear that in my head.

That night Mom and I went out for some Thai food. It was nice spending time with her before Theresa and Madeline got home. They arrived the next day, which was also my last day at work. I said my goodbyes to everyone and told them that I'd see them in two weeks, as I'd always been a quick healer. We spent Wednesday, the day before my surgery, as a family. That night, after we put Madeline to bed, Theresa and I got my belongings organized. We wanted to make sure that I had everything I needed and that we didn't bring anything unnecessary with us. We told Mom that we wanted her to stay home with Madeline, which we knew would be a challenge for her; she really wanted to be with me. But that wasn't the plan. We also didn't want Madeline to see me in the hospital. Finally, we went to bed, but neither Theresa nor I slept. I talked about our life, our baby that was on the way, and a little bit about how nervous I was. Theresa listened and talked too, but if she was anxious, she didn't show it. In fact, at no point all along had she shown any nervousness.

We were up early the next morning; the surgery was scheduled for 8:00 a.m. Theresa and I took the long walk up to the surgical area. We checked in with the nurse and then were sent to a room where some of the preparation would take place. I was weighed, had my blood pressure checked, and was handed a very large gown. I know I'm a big guy, but still, that gown was *huge*. I put it on, along with the stockings to prevent clots, the cap, and the little booties. Nothing makes a guy feel manlier than booties.

Next came the part that would become my favorite: insertion of the IV. I'd never had an IV before. It's a pretty thick needle, and as it turns out, the Acromegaly had made my skin pretty thick as well. It took them four tries before they finally got it in place. Then I was told to relax until they brought me to the next pre-op waiting room. Theresa broke the tension with her favorite joke. Actually, it is her only joke.

"Knock-knock," she said.

"Who's there?" I responded.

"Interrupting cow."

"Interrupting—"

"MOO!!!" That became our go-to joke when things get stressful.

My dad, veteran of seventeen surgeries, tells me that all ORs look the same. This one had the usual: nurses, extra surgeons, and in the corner, a guy who called himself my photographer. I made a joke about my huge gown, and the nurse pointed out that it was on inside-out. We all laughed, and I told my "photographer" to try and make me look good. He promised to do his best. I lay back, started counting backwards, ten . . . nine . . . eight . . .

And I was awake! But very uncomfortable. Dr. Flangas was standing there, and he asked me to tell him how many fingers he was holding up. It was two, but all I could think about was that I wanted Theresa next to me. I eventually answered, and then I noticed that I couldn't turn my head. The neck brace was doing its job! When I asked what time it was, Dr. Flangas told me that it was after one o' clock in the afternoon. The surgery had taken about two hours longer than it was supposed to! He explained that the veins in my neck where thicker than my thumb (and since I have Acromegaly,

I have seriously thick thumbs), and he had had to take more time to get in and out. When I asked him why, he responded simply, "Acromegaly." God I love that guy!

I had a rough night's sleep, and as I've since learned, no one sleeps well in the hospital. The next morning Dr. Flangas walked in to check on me. He asked how I was feeling, to which I succinctly replied, "Like hell." He instructed me to remove the brace and turn my head from side to side. The face I made must have indicated that I thought he was quite insane with this instruction. But, I did it, and I was surprised at how easily my head turned. He also explained that while the football injury had started the damage in my neck, the Acromegaly made things worse. Then he said words I never expected to hear—"Do you want to go home?"

"WHAT???" I asked, obviously maintaining my composure.

He said, "Feel like hell here, or at home. Which would you prefer?"

"Home," I croaked. Two hours later I was wheeled to the front of the hospital and helped into Theresa's car.

For four days I was able to eat nothing but vanilla yogurt. I lost fifteen pounds, which was fine with me. I've never been skinny. Around the same time, Gwenivere, the dog that had been with Theresa and me during our entire relationship, took a turn for the worse. One week after my surgery, we called a vet and took her over. They said there were some medications we could try, but even they sensed that Gwenie was at her end. We said we wanted to put her down. I said that I would stay in the room for it as Theresa went out to the car, unable to control her sobs. I had never had to put a dog to sleep before, and it is one of the most painful experiences I've ever had. As I felt her go limp in my arms, I ripped my neck brace off and looked down, against Dr. Flangas's orders. I held her and cried. The Valium didn't do anything to dull the pain. I eventually left the room, paid the bill (you should do this first, if you can), and got in the car with Theresa. I was carrying Gwenivere's leash, which set Theresa off again. By then I had put the neck brace back on, and we sat in the car crying. Once again I thought, "Two thousand eight can go screw itself." The running tally now: Theresa in the hospital to start the year, a brain tumor, the possibility of my company going bankrupt, neck surgery, and now our dog dying. Oh, and I still had brain surgery to look forward to!

The next week passed uneventfully. Mom went home. I was doing just fine. I still needed two naps a day, but Theresa could handle everything. Thirteen days after the surgery, we went to see Dr. Flangas. I passed all my tests and asked if I could go back to work. He asked me if I *really* wanted to. He has a very dry sense of humor. I said yes, but I did like staying home with the girls.

The next morning I got up, got dressed, and went to work. No one expected me back so soon. Well, no one but Mark. The looks of surprise were worth it. Of course, at this point almost everyone thought that this was my only surgery. But I was happy to pretend. The company was still on rocky footing, and it was a few days after my return that the president and the CEO (my friend who had brought me to the company) got into a fistfight. This has no medical relevance, except that I had to stop before I tried to break things up because I still wasn't supposed to lift anything weighing more than 5 pounds, and the president of the company was a solid 325. Thankfully, Mark had the situation under control by the time I got there. This altercation led to Mark taking over the company at the request of the board, eventually firing the CEO and the president and doing everything he needed to keep the company running. For me, this meant smooth sailing as long as I did my job. With more medical bills on the horizon, this was welcome news in a very long year.

* * *

Theresa had a Caesarian planned for August 14—still in 2008. We were incredibly excited. We knew that six weeks after that, I would have my tumor removed, but that didn't dampen our spirits at all. In fact, we felt incredibly blessed. I had excellent doctors between Dr. Flangas and Jacques. My endocrinologist also seemed terrific, but I hadn't spent much time with him yet. During one of my two visits, he brought some resident doctors in to look at me. Acromegalics are the rock stars of the endocrinology field, given how rare the disorder is. And Theresa's doctor was one of the best OBs ever. Obviously our grading is subjective, but still, we felt that we were in good hands.

Once again we had family come in to help. This time it was Theresa's mom. She came in the day before the C-section. We went to the Olive Garden for dinner. You want a woman who is nine months pregnant to get a full meal before surgery after all. After dinner, we went home, put Madeline to bed, and got Theresa prepped. Once we were ready for the next morning, Theresa and her mom sat on the couch and talked while I played some golf on the Wii. They made fun of my swing, and we all had a nice time. We were nervous, but loose, if that makes sense. Nobody slept much that night, but it was more about the excitement of meeting our newest family member.

Once again, we were up and at the hospital early, only this time it wasn't for me. I learned it is actually easier when I am the one being operated on, and much less frightening. I had been through a C-section with Theresa before; that was how Madeline was born, and an emergency C-section at that. But I had forgotten what that fear feels like, and I was facing the reminder on this day. My deepest, darkest fears have nothing to do with something bad happening to me; they always revolve around something happening to my family. We went back to the OR, and they took Theresa back to get her ready. I dressed in my scrubs, and Theresa's doctor came by to say hello. He's a naturally happy guy and was in fine spirits, seemingly as excited to meet Amelia as we were.

I was brought in to the operating room, and took my spot at Theresa's head. She had a spinal tap instead of an epidural this time and was feeling *nothing*. Last time they had to knock her out because she said that she could feel the surgery. This time, they had been working on her for five minutes when she asked, "When are you starting?" We all laughed when the doctor explained that he was almost ready to extricate the baby. It's amazing how violent a C-section actually is; I was watching one of the doctors basically jump on Theresa's chest and start pushing. Finally, we heard a cry, and Dr. Martin called me. Against strict orders from Theresa, I looked over the curtain and saw Amelia's beautiful head. Thankfully, all I saw was the baby; I had no desire to see what the inside of my wife looked like. I thought it was great that she wasn't even out and she was already crying! "Good girl," I thought.

Dr. Martin finished up. I saw Amelia wiped, measured and weighed. Then we brought the baby over so Theresa could see her. I heard her heart rate increase on the monitor as Amelia got closer to her. I took a quick picture of the two of them, but then it was time to get Amelia to the nursery. I checked one last time with Theresa to make sure that I should stick with the baby and not with her. She told me to go with Amelia, as I expected. Theresa is very paranoid about a baby switch. She watches too much television, I guess.

I watched as the nurses finished cleaning her and took more measurements. When everything seemed under control, I went back to check on Theresa. She was in bed, in a room. When I returned to the nursery, Amelia didn't look quite right. Her skin color wasn't the nice pink you expect from a newborn. The nurses were working on her, and we noticed that she wasn't maintaining her oxygen saturation. I've watched enough medical shows, so I know that when things start going wrong, the people that freak out get kicked out. I kept my mouth shut and melted into the wall while the professionals did their job. When things calmed down I simply said, "Now, I need to know what is going on." Amelia was in respiratory distress; they thought she had inhaled some fluid before finally making it out of the womb.

It would be four days before we got to hold Amelia. When one of my nieces heard about the problems, she said to my mom, "Can't they catch a break?" For a while, it was hard to tell where the monitors and leads ended and the baby began. One of us made sure to be there every three hours to give Amelia her feeding. We became close with the NICU nurses, and I have to say, they were the most wonderful people I've ever met and didn't marry. Twelve days later we brought her home. It was two days before Theresa's mom was due to leave. We dressed Madeline in a shirt that said *Big Sister*. Amelia wore a matching onesie that said *Little Sister*. Mark came over and we celebrated a bit. We were one step closer to a normal life. One unexpected hurdle cleared; one to go.

I never stopped working during this ordeal, slipping out to feed Amelia when I could. When it was behind us and she was home,

Mark came in and gave my co-worker and me some bad news. He said that the company was going down, and it was time to find another job. We had some time, but he didn't see us pulling it off. My co-worker was able to fall back on his old career, fishing for tuna in the South Pacific. I, on the other hand, had a brain tumor that was being removed in a month. I was unemployable anywhere else. Who would hire me?

Over the next month, which was all the time left until my surgery, I went about keeping my job while trying to find another one. I also cashed out my IRA to pay the mounting medical bills. I had a few appointments with Dr. Flangas, Jacques, and my endocrinologist along the way as we prepped for the surgery. My endo explained to me that if I lost any pituitary function, there was a pill for that. Interestingly, I had to urge Dr. Flangas to run through the risks this time. He actually seemed like he wanted to avoid it. The list was longer than before the last surgery.

To settle my nerves and feel like I was covering my family's bases, I called Theresa's dad and asked if all my girls could live with him, should things not go well. I also asked Mom and Dad to pay for a funeral if I needed one. Between the company's financial difficulties and all of the medical bills, we had blown through our savings, and as I mentioned before, we didn't have life insurance . . . because I was an idiot.

The pressure and stress were mounting, and we were doing our best to make sure that the pressure created a diamond out of us. But Theresa and I were bickering about the silliest things. Mom and Dad were on their way, though; this surgery was big enough to warrant both of them.

* * *

With two days to go, I went to work. Again, I was taking a day to be with the family. I went around to everyone saying, "See you in a month." Many were surprised because they had no idea about my medical issues. I had kept it quiet. I also sent an e-mail to my friends, letting them know what was happening. I hadn't told them either. Like I said earlier, I didn't want this to become the focus in my dealings with people. I made an exception when some old friends had visited earlier in the year, and I told one of them about what was going on. I asked her not to tell everyone with us until I had left for the night. Based on her reaction, I knew that it would change the tone of the evening for everyone, and what good would that do? It would have ruined a great night in Las Vegas for them, and it wouldn't have solved anything. But I sent the e-mail because if anything went wrong, I didn't want anyone blindsided.

The day before was typical, I guess . . . at least, for a day before brain surgery. I talked to every one of my siblings and my nieces and nephews. That night we went to the Olive Garden again. It has become a pre-operation tradition in the family! The surgery wasn't until three o' clock in the afternoon, so I filled up on breadsticks, soup, and all-you-can-eat pasta. We discussed our strategy for the next day. Theresa, Dad, Amelia, and I would go to the hospital. Mom would stay with Madeline. Mom is great in a crisis, but Madeline needed her more. If visiting hours allowed, Mom would see me that night.

Everyone went home with leftovers. At midnight I went downstairs and ate another plate. I knew it would be a while before I ate again. I crawled back into bed around 2:00 a.m. Everyone was sleeping pretty soundly; I was jealous. I stared at the ceiling and wondered if it was my last night. I fed the baby her middle of the night meal, staring at this beautiful being that Theresa and I had created, wondering if this would be the last meal I would give her. I needed to get this surgery done with; my mental state was shaky at best. Dr. Flangas had never lost a patient, but statistics are irrelevant if you are the outlier.

The next morning I checked our voicemail. There was a message from the anesthesiologist telling me that if I wanted, I could have a big breakfast, but no later than 6:00 a.m. I had binged on the Olive Garden food thinking that I couldn't eat at all. But I found out at 10:00 a.m. that I could've eaten. Ah well, too late now.

We left for the hospital at 11:00 a.m. I had to get a CAT scan before the surgery. We checked in and got the scan, and I went up to the surgical area. I checked in with the same nurse from last time, making a joke about being a frequent flyer. I then went to the same room as last time to get all the other pre-op work done. But the room was busier this time—SRO as they say on Broadway.

Finally, I got a seat. I spoke for a while with an older gentleman who had an abscess in his jaw that required surgery. He was older and needed to talk, so I mostly nodded along. Eventually, he asked me what I was in for. I told him I was having a tumor removed. He asked where, and I told him my head. He was quite shocked. Then Dr. Flangas and Jacques walked into the room. I got the feeling that surgeons don't often poke their heads in there. There was some light banter as they tried to dull the edge for me. I asked Dr. Flangas if he could give me a British accent while he was in my head, but he declined. The older gentleman enjoyed meeting both of my doctors and wished me luck as I was taken to the next room to get my booties, gown, leggings, etc.

This IV went worse than the first one. I had shaved most of my arm that morning, remembering the pain of removing tape from my very hairy arms. Sadly, it was in vein . . . I mean, in vain. The only vein they could get to was on a part of my arm that hadn't been shaved. Again, I was rolled to the pre-op waiting room.

Theresa spent her time with me while Dad hung out with Amelia. There were no jokes this time; we weren't feeling very funny. The anesthesiologist came by and put an anti-nausea patch behind my ear. He also put something into my IV to calm me down. It really didn't work. Theresa went and got Dad so he could see me before I went in. I rarely see him show weakness, but on this day I could see that he was shaken. We talked for a while, he told me how proud he was of how I had handled what he considered an impossible situation, and then he left, sending Theresa back in.

While we waited, I saw Dr. Flangas. He introduced me to the ear, nose, and throat doctor who would do the approach to the tumor. We said our hellos, and then I was told that the surgery was pushed back a little. There was a bit of a delay. I've wondered how that happens, but then again, my neck surgery went two hours too long, right?

Finally, the moment arrived. The bed started rolling. Theresa kissed me and told me she'd see me soon. I went into a different operating room this time; it seemed bigger and the layout was different. I moved over to the table and said hello to Dr. Flangas. Again, I made some terrible jokes. And then . . . nothing. No counting, no warning, I was put out. It's amazing, really, that we can do this to people, just knock them out and bring them back.

Hours later, I guess, I heard murmuring. I felt like hell, frankly. A million times worse than after the last surgery. But, to feel that bad, I had to be alive! Small victories, right? I struggled to open my eyes, and there was my guardian angel, Dr. Flangas. He asked me how many fingers he was holding up. "This again?" I thought. I found that I couldn't talk. I held up two fingers to prove that I could see. The concern was that the optic nerve could sustain damage during the surgery since it passed right by the tumor. I shut my eyes again. The next time I opened them, Theresa was standing there, crying.

"Is it okay to cry now?" she asked. I hadn't seen her break down a single time during our ordeal. She told me later that she cried all the time in private, but wanted to stay strong for me.

I croaked at her, "I'm ready to go home now." Obviously no one was going to let that happen. I saw Dad standing there as well. No tears, but clearly relieved. Knowing I was okay, they finally went home.

I had never been so uncomfortable in all my life. I felt like I had to urinate, badly, but there was a catheter in me. I was freezing, yet sweaty. My two front teeth felt like they had been hit with a hammer. My face was swollen; I had another IV in my right arm, an arterial line joining the IV feed in my left arm; and every few seconds the leggings inflated and deflated. Around 1:00 a.m., I was wheeled to my room in the ICU. I was special and got the ICU this time; it was very exciting.

I was still incredibly uncomfortable. (I know I'm repeating myself, but seriously! Who invented the catheter?) I couldn't breathe through my nose, so a film that felt at least a foot thick was growing on the roof of my mouth. I slowly became more aware of what I was feeling, and not much of it was pleasant. There were splints sown into my nose, I was horribly thirsty, and the catheter was *really* uncomfortable. I slept horribly, but again that's normal when one is a guest in a hospital.

Fitfully, I made it through the night. I drifted in and out of consciousness. Sometime in the morning I was taken to get another CAT scan. The techs enjoyed me. They said that usually their patients didn't talk much or help. The scan was over quickly, and back to the room I went. Jacques stopped by and told me to take it easy, and not to try and rush home. He also said that he had reviewed the surgical notes, and it looked like things had gone well. Following my own path and sticking with Dr. Flangas instead of going to a major medical center like Mom wanted was looking better and better. He also said I was in the place to be, and to relax and heal.

After Jacques left, I fell asleep again. I heard a noise a little later and opened my eyes. Mom and Dad had walked in. Mom took one look at me, started crying, and walked out to compose herself. When she came back in, she lied and told me how good I looked. She and Dad (he told me I looked like crap . . . Dad is pretty awesome) hung around for a while, but they knew that Theresa wanted to come back. When I fell asleep again, they left. I woke back up when Theresa came in. She helped me get some of the funk out of my mouth. I tried to drink something, but I couldn't use a straw: it created a horrible vacuum in my head. Having someone go into your head through your mouth, then your sinuses, only to penetrate the base of your brain does some strange things, and limiting your straw use is one of them. Also, it turned out that I had a deviated septum in my nose, but when Dr. ENT put my nose back in place (that's right), he straightened it out for me, free of charge.

Three days later, on Sunday, I got to go home. I was feeling pretty good all things considered. I spent the next month recuperating, spending time with the family, napping and drinking Slurpees. I did go to see Dr. ENT to have the splints removed, only to see that they were about seven inches long. When he pulled them out of my nose, it seemed like they would never end. Then he vacuumed out my sinuses. My face actually felt hollow; it was very strange. After that I was able to drink through a straw, which was nice. Things were looking better already.

* * *

I was very blessed. I had a slight complication with diabetes insipidus. This caused an insatiable thirst as well as chronic urination. If you've seen *A League of Their Own,* in the beginning when Tom Hanks's character meets the team, he stumbles to a trough and urinates for at least two minutes. That is what happened to me, only it happened every hour. Luckily, there is a medication for that, and it has since gone away.

I went back to work exactly four weeks after the surgery; in fact, I went back a week too early. But we had made it. I was alive, and it looked like I was tumor free. Work was still uncertain, but who cares? When I left, I wasn't sure that there would be a company to return to, but thankfully, there was. I walked back in to hugs and kind words. It was wonderful. The company still went out of business, but it lasted another year from that day.

I also got some blood work done and another MRI. When I went to have a follow-up with Dr. Flangas, he looked at the MRI results and could see no sign of the tumor. He explained that he cut out as much as he could, and when he saw a small piece touching my carotid artery, he "nuked the crap out of it." He then called in to find out my blood work results. All of my levels came back well within the normal range. My growth hormone was no longer eight times the normal amount. I shook his hand and offered my eternal gratitude, and Madeline thanked him for saving her daddy. Dr. Flangas had only operated on growth hormone–secreting tumors three times before mine. He had gotten a "total cure" on two out of the three. The actual success rate is typically thirty to forty percent for "total cures" of this type of tumor. I said, "Looks like you're at seventy-five percent!" You could tell he was pleased, but he never would have admitted it.

I've come a long way since 2008. I look back at it as the best and worst year of my life. My journey to Acromegaly was unique, as is everyone's. I now am grateful for the football injury that I had once cursed. Amelia is happy and healthy. Madeline is wonderful, and Theresa and I are stronger for the experience. We know that the tumor could come back one day, but we beat it once and are confident that things will work out in the long run. How could we not? The early diagnosis had already saved me years of life.

I also learned that near-death experiences have an expiration date. I've always loved life but could, like most other people, take it for granted. For the first six months after the surgery, small things never bothered me; I was just happy to be alive. But eventually, if you don't pay attention, you return to your old habits. Now I have to remind myself about how lucky I am, no matter the challenges. I am, and I do, every day.

Michael T. Carroll lives in San Antonio, Texas, with his wife, Theresa, and two daughters, Madeline and Amelia. He and his family happily settled in Texas after living in Florida, New York, California, North Carolina, and Nevada. He has an MBA in Financial Management from Pace University in New York and a Master's in Accountancy from the University of Phoenix.

Transsphenoidal Surgery, CSF Leak

~My Story~

Ayaka Nangumo

If there is a meaning in life at all, then there must be a meaning in suffering.
—Victor Frankl

Saturday, October 17, 2009—Tokyo, Japan

I was told to read the newspaper late in the evening. What a shame, I do not subscribe to a newspaper because I read news on the Internet. I looked at the clock. It was past 9:00 p.m. The public library was already closed, and I did not want to go out to pick up a newspaper from a convenience store. I was very tired. "OK then." I turned on my laptop and went to check the day's news. One article caught my attention: "Japanese Ministry of Health, Labour, and Welfare decided that treatment of additional 11 diseases should be subsidized from public expense" (Saturday, October 17, 2009). The list of the additional eleven medical conditions included Acromegaly. "Oh gosh! Finally!!" I sighed deeply. I felt my eyes become warm, and my vision cloudy. They were happy tears.

When I was calmed down a little, I knew I would need to get documentation to be eligible for the financial support. I wanted to prepare as soon as possible, but I knew I had to be patient because the application form would not even be ready until November. Once the forms were online, I downloaded the document from the government's website and prepared to do what I needed to get coverage. Many of the questions required me to look up my test results, so the next step was to contact my doctor.

I picked up my medical chart, which I had used to file all of my test results from the year 2007. "When was the last time I opened this chart?" I wondered. I slowly opened my records. When I saw the very first page, I started thinking of many people who had supported me ever since I was diagnosed with a pituitary tumor. My first page was the report of my very first MRI. "I can't believe I actually went through all this." Only seventeen days after that MRI, and only seven days after I was given that MRI report, I was in the operating room.

Monday, March 26, 2007—Michigan, USA

I am waiting for my neuro-ophthalmologist in her office at the MSU (Michigan State University) Clinical Center. I came here two weeks ago for the first time. Everything started in January of this year. I went to see my primary physician, at the opposite side of this campus, just to get a referral to an ophthalmologist because I thought I had lost central vision. He asked me if that was really the central vision, not peripheral. He ordered several blood tests, and I thought he was crazy. "I'm complaining about vision loss, and this guy is trying to check my blood?"

I saw an ophthalmologist, but he did not find anything wrong with my eyes. This ophthalmologist referred me to another ophthalmologist, this time one who was a retina specialist. However, the same thing happened. The retina specialist told me my retina was in wonderful shape. He told me that my vision loss was either a problem with the optic nerves or something in the brain. I shivered a little at that thought, but at the same time, I felt frustrated because nobody had found anything to explain my vision loss. It had been a month since I first complained of my problem, and I was still no closer to knowing the cause of my central vision loss. He made a referral to a neuro-ophthalmologist at MSU Clinical Center for March 12.

When I went for the visual field test, I found that I actually *had* lost the peripheral vision, *not* central vision. "That's probably not an issue with the optic nerves themselves. Isn't it a brain tumor?" I wondered. Then, I became extremely scared when Dr. Y ordered a brain MRI. Was this a tumor? The MRI result seemed to confirm my dreaded fear. I received a phone call on the twentieth because they found something. I felt a little relief and fear at the same time. I felt relieved because, finally, I would know my diagnosis. However, I was scared because now I knew something was definitely wrong with my brain. On the next day, I talked about this matter after our church choir rehearsal. Because I was an international student, I did not have a family here, and the other choir members were like a real family for me. Linn, who was in the same section as I, came to talk to me after I finished talking about the phone call from the neuro-ophthalmologist.

"I will take you to doctors' appointments, and if you would like, I will go to see the doctor with you," she said. I had been overwhelmed by that time, so I thought it would be very helpful for me to go to see a doctor with Linn to receive scary news.

That morning, Linn picked me up for my appointment with Dr. Y. When was the last time I went to a doctor's appointment with somebody? Maybe when I was in elementary school? I imagined what it would be like to be there all alone. I do not think I could be that strong, so I am glad Linn was willing to offer me some help.

Soon, Dr. Y came in. I became extremely nervous. She told me that she wanted to talk with me about the MRI result.

"Isn't it a pituitary tumor?" I asked her.

"Did you see your MRI?" She looked surprised. I had searched on the Internet with the words *peripheral vision loss* in Japanese, and most of the results were about a pituitary tumor. That was why I thought mine was also a pituitary tumor.

"There is a tumor in your brain. It's benign. The tumor is compressing your optic nerves."

Oh, I see. Now, what is the next step?

"It's a tumor, and you need surgery."

Surgery!? What!?

"They usually do the surgery through the nose. I will make a referral to Lansing Neurosurgery."

While she kept talking, I could not really follow. I saw Linn pulling out a notebook, and she started writing down what the doctor was saying. My mind was racing with a million thoughts: Surgery? It's a neurosurgery? How can I do this? I read on the Internet about the neurosurgery that can be done through the nose, but wasn't it for a small tumor? How big is mine? I read that the success rate depended on the size of the tumor. Is mine big? Unfortunately, I did not actually ask any of those questions because I became quite thirsty and was not able to ask the questions I wanted to ask the most. I was very lucky to have Linn there supporting me.

After the appointment, the secretary made a referral to a neurosurgeon. I would be seeing a neurosurgeon the day after tomorrow. Then, Linn told me that I had several blood tests that needed to be done that day. I missed that information, oops! I felt so thankful that she came to the appointment with me. After I finished the blood tests, I told Linn that I wanted to know the size of my pituitary tumor. She replied, "You need to get a copy of the MRI images and the report for the neurosurgeon, and maybe it is written on the report." I missed that information, again!

We went to the radiology department to receive the copy of my MRI and the report. When they handed me the report, I started searching for numbers.

"How was it?" Linn asked.

"I think it will be OK." I was in denial. It was much bigger than I expected.

Monday, April 2, 2007—Michigan, USA

I was having a restless night, and then I realized it was already April 2. I could not believe that I was having the first surgery of my life, and what is more, it was neurosurgery. "Is it really happening? I'm in a foreign country and getting my first surgery while I'm here? What did I do wrong, Lord?" I was born in Japan, and I came to the United States to study in college when I was eighteen. It was only a week ago that I made an international call to Japan to talk to my mother. I told her that I was diagnosed with a form of brain tumor, and I was getting a surgery.

The operation was scheduled for 1:00 p.m. on Monday, April 2, 2007, in Lansing, Michigan. I was repeatedly recalling what Dr. S, my ENT surgeon, said to me: "We will take good care of you."

I was supposed to come into the hospital by 10:00 a.m. on the date of my surgery. My friend Linn came to my apartment to pick me up around 9:15 a.m. It was only about a fifteen-minute drive to the hospital from my apartment, but it felt much longer because I was thinking of the whole process of getting diagnosed and how quickly things had gone since the diagnosis was made.

I suspect my first symptom of Acromegaly was when I moved to the United States to study abroad. I was eighteen and recovering from an eating disorder. I started struggling with anorexia nervosa when I was around fifteen. A year later from the onset of anorexia, I started experiencing binge eating and purging, in my case, self-induced vomiting. Ever since, I have had a body image issue, even today. I have always felt I am bigger than I am, and I feel like I need to be a lot smaller.

With this background, it was especially hard for me to accept all the change in my appearance. First, I became a lot taller. I was 163 cm (5'4") when I finished high school in March 2001. However, when I came back to Japan in 2004, I was 169 cm (5'6½"). I also felt like I was getting bigger, but I tried to convince myself that my mind was still playing a horrible game with me. The disturbing truth was that I really was getting bigger. My chest bones got bigger, my shoulders got bigger, and my head got bigger, so I felt I was becoming fat. My hands and feet also got bigger, and I learned in a human life science class that this was also linked to Acromegaly. When I saw pictures of a lady with Acromegaly in the textbook, I felt like I saw myself because some of her facial features were quite similar to mine. But I told myself that this kind of rare disease would never happen to me.

In January 2007, as I mentioned earlier, I started asking for medical help because of the visual field abnormality. I first noticed partial vision loss in summer 2006, but I did not take any action.

However, I became very concerned at the end of 2006 because I was feeling tired and noticed I had headaches all the time too. I could not ignore these problems any longer, and that was why I started looking for answers in January 2007.

So here I am. Finally, I have received the diagnosis, and I am getting the surgery today. While Linn was still driving, I was thinking of all the doctors who had been involved until today: my general physician, two ophthalmologists, the neuro-ophthalmologist, the neurosurgeon, and the ENT surgeon. Especially after my first appointment with Dr. Y, my neuro-ophthalmologist, things became quite intense for me. I saw her on March 12 and had an MRI on March 16. On March 26, Dr. Y told me that I had a benign tumor on my pituitary, and I needed a surgery. I saw my neurosurgeon, Dr. H, and ENT surgeon, Dr. S, on March 28. They wanted to schedule on Friday, March 30, but thanks to my ENT surgeon's schedule conflict, it became Monday, April 2. I do not think I was emotionally ready on March 30, so I am glad I got two more days to get prepared. All these things had happened in such a short period of time, so it was hard for me to comprehend. However, thanks to the additional two days, I got Sunday right before my surgery date. The congregation of my church gave me a lot of positive words on that day, so I felt a lot stronger to face this scary reality to go into the operating room on the next day.

While I was still thinking about all of these memories, we got to the hospital parking lot. I was feeling a little anxious, but I was doing okay. After I signed in, they took me to my bed in the room where many other patients were waiting for their surgeries. Hospital staff came to do final testing, such as urine, blood tests, blood pressure, and heart rate. They gave me a hospital gown and a pair of stockings to prevent blood clots. They also inserted an IV in my left forearm. It was the first IV insertion of my life, and it was not as painful as I had imagined.

After all the testing, a gentleman came in and handed me the consent form. The form explained why I was getting the surgery and, of course, the risks of the surgery. He said, "If you understand and are fine with it, just put your initials." I started reading and putting initials for each statement without thinking a lot until I reached the section that explained risks. The consent stated that a cerebrospinal fluid (CSF) leak may occur as a complication of this surgery. My neurosurgeon told me about this, but I did not know much about what would happen if the leak occurred. He explained that they need to drain the CSF through the lower back, and that was the only thing I knew about it. I did not know how the fluid was going to be drained. This uncertainty gave me some fear, but I signed anyway. Then, I came to the part of the form that goes something like, "Patients may lose some/complete vision." I was getting the surgery to bring back my peripheral vision. I had a hard time accepting this statement. I started thinking about my options. "If I do not go through with this surgery, I might lose all vision. It's better to try and lose than not to try at all and lose." After I weighed costs and benefits, I signed.

Finally and inevitably, the consent stated that, in rare instances, there would be serious complications, including *death*. I stopped for awhile. I imagined what would happen if I would die in the United States, which is a foreign country for me. That would be very hard for my family, both financially and emotionally. When I read this, I understood why there are some people who cancel their surgery on the scheduled day. Going through the consent is very scary. I, personally, tried to focus on the benefits rather than the risks so that I could convince myself to get a surgery I knew I needed. However, the consent form kept asking me, basically, "Are you fine with these risks?" So, it redirected my mind to the scary side of the surgery, and my brain took note. Taking account of this, it is understandable that some patients find it too overwhelming to give consent to do the surgery. I felt fear, but when I saw Linn staying with me, I felt safe and courageous at the same time, so I took a deep breath and signed the final section.

After I had gone through the consent form, they gave me some pills with a sip of water. I found it hard to swallow them, but I managed OK. Then, they carried me to another room where I was getting the first anesthesia. While they were carrying me, I saw Dr. S, my ENT surgeon. I was anxious a bit, but as soon as I saw him, I could believe that I would be OK. "We'll take good care of you, Ayaka." I immediately recalled what he said when I saw him last week. The room was a little chilly, so I asked for more blankets. A young resident came in and introduced herself. She told me that her field was pediatrics, and she was going to observe my operation as part of the training. I felt a little happy that my surgery could contribute for education.

While I was waiting for the anesthesiologist, I looked around the room. It looked like one of the scenes of a TV medical drama. When I recognized the fact that I was actually in the scene, I started feeling nervous. I was glad Linn stayed with me all this time. I would have felt so alone without her support.

Awhile later, Dr. S came in. "Hi, Ayaka, how are you?"

I answered, "Good."

"Dr. H and I will take good care of you."

I do not remember more of what he said that time because I was quite anxious. What I do remember, though, was how he talked to me. He spoke in a way that really helped me to calm myself down. He was smiling and talked to me with confidence. When I saw him talking in this manner, I felt everything was going to be OK after all. At that point, I felt a lot of support from many people—my doctors, Linn, my best friends, all the people from the church, my parents. My heart felt so warm. "I will be OK. God will take care of everything, and Dr. H and Dr. S will do great."

The anesthesiologist came in. I do not remember his name. He asked me, "Do you know what surgery you are getting?"

I answered, "It's a transsphenoidal tumor resection."

He also asked me why I was getting the surgery.

"Because I have a tumor on my pituitary." I did not know why he was asking these questions.

After he asked these things, he started explaining about general anesthesia. He told me I was getting the first anesthesia in this room through IV and the second to put me into a deep sleep in the other room. He said that I would feel my mind go cloudy after the first administration. He told me to take off my glasses, so I did and handed them to Linn. The medication was administered from the IV injection port. Gradually, I started feeling "cloudy," as he described. They told me that they were going to take me to another room. I was under the first anesthesia, so my memory is not very clear, but I do remember I felt alone for the first time because Linn was not allowed to go into the room with me. I felt very sleepy, and I thought I fell asleep.

When I realized I was in a room with surgical lights, I wondered if that was the operating room. The staff asked me to move onto the table in the room, but I could not move very well, so they helped me. They put an anesthesia mask on my face. They asked me questions like, "Does it snow in Japan?" I answered, "Sometimes." I still remember the last question I answered because now I find it funny. "Do you have winter season in Japan?" "Sometimes . . ." I was out.

". . . Ayaka?" A lady's voice woke me up. Is it over already? What time is it? Is it still April 2? Am I really alive? Where in the hospital am I? When I woke up, the sensation was exactly the same as waking up every morning. I slowly opened my eyes, feeling tired. I did not feel any pain, but I noticed a pile of gauze taped on my nose. I decided to breathe through my mouth. Next, I felt a tube on my mouth. It was releasing a cold air, which I supposed was the oxygen.

"Ayaka?" The lady talked to me again.

I answered, "Yes."

"Oh good, now you're up. You did very well, sweetheart. Your surgery is over. Now, could you tell me your full name and your date of birth for me?"

I answered.

Then she asked me, "Do you know today's month?"

"April," I said.

The next question made me laugh a bit. "Who is the president of the United States?"

". . . Bush?" I almost said Kerry as a joke. It was a good sign that I had room for a dark humor, at least.

After the reflex and cognition test, they told me that I could go back to sleep. I felt quite tired, so I wanted to fall asleep, but I felt my blood clots were almost clogging my airway, so I asked for a small basin to spit them out. It looked quite disgusting, but I felt a lot better. Now, I started looking around. I first noticed that I was able to see better than before. It was a joy to notice that I gained back my peripheral vision. I was excited to see things on my side, especially on my right because the peripheral vision loss of my right eye was outstanding. I recalled the disturbing consent form that I read before the surgery that listed the complications, including the vision loss. "I didn't lose my vision; I gained it back. I'm glad I decided to go through this surgery."

I looked around more. Suddenly, I wondered if they had catheterized me, but I could not figure that out. Instead, I noticed that they had wrapped my legs to a machine that was massaging my legs, probably to prevent blood clots. Then, I was hooked into a heart monitor and a blood pressure monitor. My IV line was still on my left arm.

While I was looking around the recovery room, Dr. S came in.

"Hi, Ayaka. You did very well, and the surgery was a success. It was ten out of ten. When we opened, the tumor came out on its own, so it went very well. And you did great!"

"Thank you, Dr. S."

"Is your vision OK?"

"Yes, I can see just fine."

"Great! Now get some rest, OK?"

"Thank you."

We shook hands. Oh, thank you, Lord. Now, it's really over. I felt more relaxed after I talked with Dr. S, so I fell asleep for awhile.

I do not remember what time it was when they carried me to the neuro-ICU. Dr. H told me that I was going to stay in the ICU for 24 hours to be monitored, so I was not shocked or anything to be there. I do not remember when Linn came in, but I felt very thankful that she was there to stay with me during this whole time. I still do not know how many hours my surgery took, but she waited for me.

For the first several hours, I slept a lot. I was not hungry or thirsty at all. I had been actually very worried that I would become outrageously thirsty. Here is the reason why I was very concerned about the thirst. Once Dr. Y, my neuro-ophthalmologist, told me that I had a pituitary tumor and needed surgery, I had researched the pituitary surgery extensively. When I was reading other patients' experiences with transsphenoidal surgery, I remember one patient wrote about being extremely thirsty after the surgery, so I became quite worried. I can resist hunger without much problem, but I have a hard time dealing with thirst for some reason. However, the staff told me that the thirst would not be that bad since the IV would give me a lot of fluid. "You'll be all right."

Then at dinner time, my aide gave me two vanilla puddings. I did not know I was able to eat already. I was quite happy for a moment; then, I remembered I was told that I might not taste anything for several days or weeks after the transsphenoidal surgery, so I wondered if that were true. With my first spoonful of vanilla pudding, I could taste its sweetness, but because I could not smell due to the surgical damage to the sinus, I was not able to tell if it was vanilla or another flavor. I was a little disappointed and really hoped that I would be able to sense the smells again. A similar thing happened when I asked for apple juice. I tasted sweetness and sourness, but I could not tell if it were apple juice or something else.

Tuesday, April 3, 2007—CSF Leak

I tried to sleep, but I was restless. I felt a little frustrated because I was awfully tired, but I was not able to get a wink of sleep. "Well, I slept a lot today, I suppose. I slept for how many hours I don't know during the surgery." I gave up, and that was the time I fell asleep for awhile. To my surprise, I was able to breathe through my nose. As midnight passed, I woke up again because my gauze was sagging wet. I called the nurse. She changed my gauze. I felt good with new, dry gauze, so I fell asleep again. However, I was woken up by the wet gauze again and again. By 4:00 a.m., I sensed something was truly wrong. I was not able to lie down anymore because the fluid was clogging my airway. The phrase *CSF leak* came across my head. "Could you turn on the light for me, please?" I asked the nurse because I wanted to see my gauze. I thought I might be in big trouble if the gauze was not reddish brown. I looked at the pile and figured it was not blood. My nurse left the room to call Dr. H. She came back, looking very sorry. She told me that I needed to sit upright until Dr. H came in later. I felt quite weary. Why do bad things happen to me all the time? I wanted to think positively, but I was just not able to. By the time I was told to sit upright, I was very tired and sleepy, so I really wanted to lie down and fall asleep in my own bed at home with a cozy blanket. Yet, I didn't have any other choice, did I? While I was wondering what was going to happen in the next several hours, a lady came in for a blood test. After she left, I turned on the TV and waited for Dr. H for several hours.

I do not know how many hours I waited, but my neurosurgeon came in early in the morning. He told me that my CSF was leaking out, so he needed to drain the fluid from my lower back to help the healing of the dura, and the procedure was called *lumbar puncture.* The dura mater is a layer that protects the brain and spinal cord, and inside the layers, there is CSF bedding the brain. In transsphenoidal surgery, when neurosurgeons approach the surgical site, they cut the layers, then sew them back when the operation is finished. During this sewing-up process, they use a type of glue also. In this way, it's unlikely that the CSF will leak out from the layers where they cut. However, in some rare cases, the dura mater gets torn from the pressure of the CSF. In my case, the resected mass was very large, so the CSF got into where the tumor was located. The sewed-back dura was not able to take the pressure of the CSF, so the layer eventually got torn, and the CSF leaked out from the surgical site. I did not know what kind of procedure the lumbar drain was, so I felt very scared. I wished that I had asked about the procedure when the CSF leak had been mentioned as a potential complication of surgery. If I had known about it, I could have expected what would happen so that I could have been more prepared, mentally. Before the procedure, they handed me a consent form again. Dr. H told me that it would take about ten to fifteen minutes.

I was hearing my nursing assistant and the neurosurgeon discussing how they should position my body. It seemed like there were two possibilities: lie-down and sit-up. The doctor told me to sit and curl my back. He taped a surgical sheet with a hole on my back. The local anesthesia went just fine. "I can handle this!" I thought. He cut my skin, but I did not feel anything. Good! Then, he grabbed a huge needle. "Oh my! Don't tell me he is gonna poke that stuff into me. Oh please! I hope I won't feel anything." Unfortunately, the doctor told me that I would feel pressures. And for the next several minutes, I was screaming. I had never experienced that kind of pain before. When he poked some nerves with the needle, my legs and arms tingled, and the reflex was very unpleasant. And this unfamiliar type of pain was absolutely horrible. It was so painful that I could not even cry. All this time, my nurse was holding my hand tightly, with a lot of encouraging words. "You're doing great. I went through that when I had a baby, so I know it's painful. I know you can handle it." She started rubbing my upper shoulder at the same time. Slowly, the pain disappeared. "It's almost over now, Ayaka. He is taping the tube on your back." Oh, finally. Up to today, that was the worst kind of pain I have ever experienced. I have heard of other patients who did not have that much pain from this same procedure, so I suppose it is not everybody who goes through such horrible pain from the lumbar drain.

For about five minutes, I was fine. Soon, however, I started experiencing a nauseating headache that I had never experienced before. My nurse immediately injected some pain killer—I believe morphine—through the IV. Shortly after that, I started breathing fast and felt the muscle strained. For two days, I suffered from bad headaches, nausea, and vomiting. I forced myself to eat something for each meal, but I could only eat a very small amount, like several spoonfuls of mashed potato and soup. Even so, I threw up a lot because of nausea. On that day, I was holding my Bible tightly whenever I felt discouraged because of the pain. I asked my nurse why I suddenly started feeling so sick and was in unbearable pain. "The brain is embedded in a fluid. It's like water, you know. Now, we're draining the fluid from your brain to help the healing of torn dura, so basically, you're brain is very, very thirsty." The purpose of the lumbar puncture for CSF leak is to release the pressure on the torn dura. Lumbar puncture drains the CSF at a certain speed so that the CSF will not get into the surgical site to press the torn layer. As a result, the brain feels the change of intracranial pressure (pressure within the skull), and that causes the headache.

Wednesday, April 4, 2007—Panic Attack

I was feeling really horrible all day, but I do not have much memory of that day. I was asleep most of the time with the help of a lot of pain killers. I do remember I was very depressed and panicky, though. I also remember Linn came to visit me. I felt so thankful, but very sad at the same time that I was not able to talk to her much because I was very sick. When my nurse came in, I asked her, "Am I going to get well?" I wanted to cry so badly. I felt my tears coming up, but I held it in. She said, "Well, there are good days and bad days, but I believe every day is a progress." I was too afraid to ask how long it would take for me to get well or when my CSF leak would be over. I felt hopeless, and also quite anxious.

There was another thing started in my mind at the same time. After the surgery, I noticed I was catheterized, and it was a Foley catheter, not a Robinson catheter. Well, both types of catheters are inserted into the bladder to drain the urine. In order to be retained, Foley catheters have balloons, which are inflated after the insertion. Robinson catheters do not have the balloon. I could not stand the idea of a Foley catheter for some reason, and I started experiencing discomfort from the inserted catheter. It was always there, so I needed to distract myself. Also, when the angle was not right, it was not draining the urine properly, so I felt some urge to urinate, yet I was not able to do so. This was a big problem for me since that Tuesday. I had been able to manage this almost phobic-like feeling toward Foley catheter until midnight of that day. However, the problem occurred at midnight.

Linn came in, which I believe was her second time to visit me on that day. I opened my eyes, but I felt too weak to talk to her. I heard my nurse come in to do something to my lumbar drain. I also heard Linn and my nurse talking about my CSF leak. I do not remember much of their conversation, but I specifically remember Linn asked the nurse how long it would usually take to get the torn dura healed. The nurse answered, "Each case is different, but it can take about fifteen days." Fifteen? Like two weeks? Am I going to be like this for two weeks? I felt totally hopeless and disappointed. They probably did not know I was listening. I started imagining me having this terrible headache, feeling nauseous, and being immobile for two weeks. My Bible was under my blanket, so I tried to hold it tightly. "Oh, Father, help me. I cannot handle this hardship without your support."

I was not able to sleep on that day, so I was watching TV to distract myself from all the discomfort. Soon, I became very aware that my room was closed, and I was hooked up to multiple things. I started counting everything that was attached to my body, such as heart monitor, catheter, IV line, and so on. I counted thirteen lines. All of a sudden I started feeling like I was going insane. I called my nurse. By the time she came in, I was in the middle of a panic attack. "I'm wired up. I can't get out of this place. I can't move. I'm going crazy! I can't do this anymore. I'm wired up." My breathing was very fast, and I kept on saying something.

I heard my nurse talking to me with a calming voice. "Ayaka? Ayaka? Look at me. Just look at me now. You're not wired up, and you're not in an enclosed space. You're OK, sweetheart." She was trying to calm me down.

However, I started repeating those words: "I can't do this anymore. I can't do this anymore."

The nurse took out a vial from the medicine cabinet. I got scared. "Is she going to inject something? Am I going to be OK?" She came with a syringe and injected something into my IV port. It was a tranquilizer. Shortly after that, I started feeling very tired, and I fell asleep. I did not know if it was a dream or if I was hallucinating or if it really happened, but I saw a man-like figure show up with a gentle wind. He told me, "Your prayers are answered. You are healed."

Thursday, April 5, 2007—Great Progress and a Friend's Love

I woke up, and surprisingly, I did not feel too sick. My terrible headache was gone, and I started eating pretty well. When my nurse asked me how I was doing, I answered, "I'm feeling much better." I was able to smile.

"Good for you!" She smiled back. "I heard you were able to sit for awhile yesterday." Was I? Oh, yes! I actually did.

I felt too depressed to be immobile on the bed all day, and I begged my nurse to let me move around, but she gave me a very strict no. "Can I at least sit on a chair?" I was not hesitant.

"Well, if it makes you feel happier, we can help you."

When I sat on the chair, my headache got so much worse, but emotionally, I felt less miserable. I felt, "See? I can sit, just like normal people." Also, by sitting on the chair, I could distract myself from the discomfort of the Foley. I thought it was a dream, but it seems like it actually happened.

Because I had been doing so poorly the past two days, Linn brought steamed brown rice and white rice with miso soup. I could not believe she actually did so much for me. I heard she asked several people what Japanese people want to eat when they feel sick. To be honest, eating non-Japanese food was not really appetizing for me. I had wished to have a good old Japanese sick meal, something like *okayu,* which is salty rice porridge, and some miso soup, so I was very thankful that she brought Japanese food for me. When I put the food into my mouth, tears flowed from my eyes. I felt her love and support. I also was very thankful to God for giving me such a wonderful friend.

In the early evening, the nursing assistant came and told me that I should start walking. I was very excited. I needed to walk with the IV stand, carrying a bunch of things. "Move slowly, hon." When I sat upright, I felt lightheaded a little. I slowly stood up with help. I felt even more lightheaded. Gradually, however, I felt just fine, so I started walking with assistance. I was only allowed to walk around in the neuro-ICU, but I was so happy that I did not have to be in my hospital room all day anymore.

Friday, April 6, 2007—Discharge

Dr. H came in the morning to check how my CSF leak was doing. I did not feel salty water running in the back of my throat anymore. All this time I thought I had tasted salty water because of a runny nose, but as it turns out, it was my CSF.

Dr. H told me I might be able to go home that day.

"Really?" I asked him, all excited.

"And once you get discharged, make sure you see an endo. Your tumor was positive for growth hormone and something else." I should see who? Endo? What is that? Well, I'll ask this later. There should be some explanation when I get discharged.

After he left, I asked my aide, "Could you remove my catheter for me as soon as possible?" I was begging. She came back with several items, and they removed my Foley. I felt great. "Oh, finally! It's out! No more!!"

They told me that my lumbar drain should be removed soon. I tried to see my tube for the drain (lumbar puncture), and it looked like a tail coming out from my lower back. I giggled. "This looks funny! I've got a tail!" My IV site was painful too, so I wanted it to be removed, but they told me I needed to wait. After I ate my lunch, I got my official discharge from the hospital. My nurse came to remove my lumbar drain and the IV. Then, she started giving me discharge information: follow-ups, when to call doctors, and what kind of activity I should avoid. She told me that I should do follow-ups with an endocrinologist. I had no idea what an *endocrinologist* was. I had no idea how to pronounce this word, even. At least, I knew endocrinologist was some kind of doctor because the word ended with *-ologist*. She told me to call my general practitioner first to get a referral.

Some "Should-Haves"

When I think back how I went through the surgery, there were many "should-haves."

First, I wish I had brought a pen and a notebook (or at least some paper to write on) to the medical appointments from the beginning. I did not know taking notes during an appointment was essential. I still bitterly remember my second appointment with Dr. Y. Thanks to Linn, who took notes for me, I did not miss important information while the doctor was telling me about the diagnosis, surgery, and testing that I needed to complete before the surgery. If I had been ready to take notes, I do not think I would have felt too overwhelmed to focus on the important information she was giving me. I learned from this experience, so now I take notes during each medical appointment. In this way, I can read them back later to know what is going on in my body and what kind of medication the doctor is prescribing for which conditions.

Second, and this is related to the first one, I wish I had asked all the questions that I had. For instance, as you see, I did not ask my neurosurgeon enough questions about a possible CSF leak. I now know that uncertainty gave me a lot of fear. If I had known what would be done if the CSF leak happened, I do not think I would have been as fearful because I would have known what to expect. I wish I had written down my questions and concerns before each appointment to minimize the worry. After the discharge from the hospital, I started writing down all the questions in my "medical appointment notebook" so that I do not forget to ask everything that I want to know about my conditions and treatments.

Third, I wish I had sought medical help much earlier. If I did, my tumor might not have grown that big. I noticed something was slightly wrong about five years before the diagnosis was made. Acromegaly can cause many complications, and I have several. If I had started seeing doctors earlier, the diagnosis could have been made earlier; the surgery could have been done earlier; and I would have had fewer complications. Now, when I feel something wrong with my body, I tell my doctor during the monthly follow-ups.

After the Very Last Page

My discharge instruction paper was the very last page of the folder named *Surgery* in my personal medical chart. However, my battle with Acromegaly did not end there. Until I requested my pathology report, I did not know my tumor was producing growth hormone. Also, the report said my tumor cells were an aggressive kind. When I saw my endocrinologist for the first time, he ordered countless cancer screening tests, including a colonoscopy. Then, he decided to start me on Sandostatin LAR (20 mg), but I faced financial issues because this medication was extremely expensive. Thanks to Novartis's PAP (Patient Assistance Program), I was able to receive it for free while I was in the United States, but I admit that I spent many days crying because I thought I would not be able to receive any treatment. From all the stress of dealing with Acromegaly while I was far away from my home across the ocean, I started struggling from clinical depression at the same time. However, I do not feel that I am the unlucky one. I truly feel blessed to go through such a rough time because I gained a lot from this experience.

Through this experience, first, I have gained a lot of medical knowledge. For instance, I can name all the pituitary hormones, both anterior and posterior. Not limited to hormones, I gained knowledge about human anatomy and physiology. I learned a lot about medications. I also had many chances to learn about different kinds of diseases and how people with these conditions are coping.

Second, I have built even stronger friendships. At the same time, now I know who my true friends are. While I was in the neuro-ICU, there was no day that I did not receive a greeting card. I felt truly blessed to have such wonderful friends. Linn physically stayed with me during my hardest time. I have not yet mentioned my pastor John-Ross; my friend Anna, who was also fighting her own brain tumor with radiotherapy; several choir members from the church; and Amaka and Ramzi, who are all the people who visited me while I was in the ICU. There were many people who prayed for me. When I saw all the get-well cards, I felt the kindness and love of all these people. Moreover, I met many wonderful individuals through patient support groups internationally. Each member of these support groups is a hero and also has been a great support to me.

Finally, I learned to feel others' pain. This is something you need to earn from your own experience, so I think all these medical challenges are a gift for my personal growth. When I listen to others' challenges and problems they are facing, I have learned to put myself in their shoes. I have suffered greatly with Acromegaly, with surgery, a CSF leak, financing medications, and so on; but when I think of all the gains, it was not necessarily an unfortunate experience for me.

Tuesday, December 1, 2009

While I was filling out the application form for the medical expense subsidy, there were many thoughts that came into my mind. What I have gone through, how my life has changed ever since the surgery, and what I have gained from this medical condition. When I finished filling out the form and closed the chart, I could not help but sigh deeply. "That whole week—the week I had my operation—was really unforgettable." I brought the paper to my endocrinologist to have her complete the application form on November 19. Today, December 1, 2009, each prefecture (that's like a state in the US) started accepting the subsidy application forms from the patients with the additional eleven medical conditions. Today was a very special day for me, and I am sure it was so for other patients. We finally made a big step forward for better quality of life for patients who are living with Acromegaly. When I came back from work today, I opened my chart again to see all the records that are related to the surgery. When I saw my discharge instructions from the hospital, I closed the file. Then, I grabbed the next chart: the medical record from my current hospital in Japan. Now, my surgery is over, we have gained more patients' rights here in Japan, and my/our battle still continues.

Ayaka Nangumo was born in Japan in 1983 and currently resides in Tokyo. She lived in the United States for seven years to study psychology (2001-2008). She was diagnosed with Acromegaly while she was working as a research assistant in Michigan State University, where she received her Bachelor's degree in Psychology. She went through surgery when she was in this foreign country, and it was a great success. Her plan after the surgery was to finish her Master's degree at Ball State University. However, her hardships (the health concerns, the medical expenses, and the psychological distress) eventually brought her back home to Japan in 2008. Although she was weary at first, she started to take action to link Japanese patients to patients in other parts of the world because she felt Japanese patients were isolated from the world due to the language barrier. The progress is slower than she wishes, yet she is patiently making an effort.

Radiotherapy

Tyson Koerper

I've never known anybody to achieve anything without overcoming adversity.
—Lou Holtz

My name is Tyson Koerper. I was diagnosed with Acromegaly in 2006. Upon learning that I had this disease, I underwent a partially successful surgery and was subsequently put on medication to lower my growth hormone (GH) levels. Upon incomplete remission of the disease, I opted for radiotherapy in an effort to eventually normalize my GH levels and prevent my tumor from continuing to grow. What follows is my story, told as best I can, about what it was like in the early stages through to today. I will put an extra emphasis on the unique experience of undergoing radiation treatment for this disease, what to expect, and how to cope. Along the way, I would like the reader to hopefully see things in my story that are reflections of things from either their own story or that of a loved one: the fear, hope, support, confusion, and eventual victory over this disease. If the reader is not quite at that victory stage, the most important thing I can hope someone would walk away from my story with is that with a little patience and support, you'll get there.

At twenty-six years old, I was working full time in my chosen field as a graphic designer—the field in which I had recently earned my degree. My then-fiancée and I were living together in a small apartment, enjoying our time together as young adults in eager pursuit of our future goals. We worked hard, but had enough free time to go out and enjoy ourselves, and even build some savings. Relatively speaking, life was good. But despite my overall satisfaction with the positive direction of things, I was feeling some growing tension to take my career to a higher level. After all, it had been three years since I took my first job directly out of college; and the feeling of moving onward and upward began tugging at the back of my mind. My projects began to feel more and more routine, and deadlines loomed as motivation sank. I was coming to a crossroads in life where I felt I had other places to be, more to learn, and a foundation for my future still to establish. I began making a strong effort to expand my design portfolio and tighten my résumé. I was ready to begin making strides towards a greener pasture.

During this time, however, there was an almost unconscious feeling that something was awry. Call it a premonition if you will, but looking back on where this unease was coming from, there were things that I had taken note of in my pre-diagnosis days that were later attributable to an underlying issue, unknown to me or anyone at the time. The slow progression of an underbite over the past several years, night sweats, mood swings, loss of energy, puffy hands, puffy face, jaw pain, headaches, depression—all possible effects of excessive human growth hormone or a growing pituitary tumor. The symptoms were so subtle in their development that many were attributable to other causes; symptoms that were relatively harmless individually, and seemingly unrelated. To connect all of the dots would have been difficult for most doctors, and almost impossible for me. I naively attributed my problems to stress and aging. I have a way of sweeping things under the rug, and that's exactly what I was doing. Denial? Maybe. But I would say that it was more of a naïveté that the normal course of aging shouldn't involve so many strange symptoms. Thus goes the story of the majority of Acromegaly sufferers.

So I ignored my symptoms and retained my focus on career advancement at all costs. I committed myself fully to the pursuit of new employment. I spent long hours late into the night expanding my portfolio outside of my full-time job, sending my résumé to prospective employers, and self-teaching new skills. I was able to land a few jobs here and there as a freelancer, which I considered progress, so I pressed on and worked with diligence. A couple of the side jobs I had picked up turned into lucrative business relationships, and things finally started to pay off in the summer of 2006 when one of the advertising agencies I had been freelancing for extended an offer to come aboard full-time. This was the opportunity I had been waiting for. I was offered this position over several other candidates, and the type of work I was doing was exactly the type of work I had been dreaming of—designing magazine advertisements for the motorsports industry. I was once again enthusiastic about my career, and after resigning from my then-present job, I began working for the new agency two weeks later.

Like any new job, the break-in period was quite stressful, and if you know anything about advertising, the lightning-fast pace combined with the constant deadlines and long hours can make learning a new position all the more nerve-wracking. This was different, though, and something inside me knew it. By the end of the first week, I vividly recall a meltdown at my apartment in which I confessed to my fiancée that I may have made a very big mistake. I felt that I had given up a rather comfortable job for what I began to feel was a job I couldn't handle, mentally or physically. She reassured me that being the new guy and learning the ropes was always difficult and that walking away would be a defeatist's attitude. This encouragement got me through the next couple of days.

By week two, the words of encouragement began to wear off. I was stressed to the point of exhaustion, every day. I was burned out, not from just the new job and its demanding nature, but from weeks and months of built-up anticipation over that very same new job. All the tension, worry, enthusiasm, and few periods of rest finally caught up with me. The nearly subconscious concern over my headaches, depression, swollen hands, jaw pain, and fatigue began to stir itself more and more with my current work stresses. In times of distress, I have an awful habit of allowing myself to focus on thinking of only the negative while ignoring anything positive. This was no different, and the stress of my new work looking more like a mistake meshed right in there with all the other slight oddities I noticed in myself.

I've always been a level-headed individual, but I couldn't help but think that in some way I was slowly losing my grip on things.

So by this time, I really began to think that something might be very wrong, either with my body or my mind. I was three weeks into the new position that I had worked so hard to get to. It was as close to a dream job as I could have imagined at the time; and my personal life had been humming along wonderfully. While I should have been grinning ear to ear with pride and enthusiasm, the opposite was true. I began to feel awful, all the time. The stress of a new career and the long hours the new job demanded had exacerbated my still-unknown underlying condition. I was nearly immobile with anxiety and depression. My headaches banded together to form one constant headache, and I had very little energy. I was waking up every night in sweat-drenched sheets, popping Advil like candy, and dragging myself around just to accomplish menial tasks. Productivity at work tanked, pulling me into an even greater downward spiral of anxiety over fears my new employer would take issue with my performance level. I had to ask myself why I felt the way I did. What the hell was wrong with me?

Just when I was making a decision to seek help for my emotional problems, a new and more urgent symptom emerged, which, as a graphic artist, caused immediate alarm. The left side of my peripheral vision began to diminish, rapidly. As I would come to learn, a growing pituitary tumor can press against optic nerves, causing a condition known as bitemporal hemianopia, in which the left and right periphery diminish so slowly that, often, the sufferer will not realize for some time. But in my case, the loss of vision in my left eye seemed drastic. At this time, I was still in a bit of denial and assumed my eye issue was either a burst vessel from all the stress or something temporary that would just go away on its own. However, with some hesitation and at the strong urging of my fiancée's father, who was actually a medical doctor, I made an appointment with an ophthalmologist. I withheld an alarmist's attitude by thinking I was doing this to simply rule out the serious stuff. "There's nothing wrong with me; I'm perfectly healthy!" I told myself, "Nothing to worry about, just run through the tests and let the doc tell me what I already know." As it would soon turn out, though, it was this budding issue in my left eye that would be the straw that broke the camel's back and that would lead to my ultimate diagnosis.

My diagnosis wasn't sudden. I first made the appointment with the eye doctor, and after a battery of tests, I was informed that this issue had nothing to do with my eye itself; rather, it was something neurological. The "differential diagnosis" on my initial report included stroke, brain lesion, and optic neuritis (a presenting symptom of multiple sclerosis); and God knows what else was on that set of notes. I tried to hide my deep fears of the worst scenarios from my fiancée, but it was evident that I was troubled by what looked to be emerging evidence of something serious. My fiancée and I agreed that since the situation was in limbo for the time being, we would focus attention on our usual routine of enjoying the small pleasures we could afford. My next appointment was with a neurologist. Again, a battery of tests still wasn't pointing to an obvious diagnosis. The next logical step was to have an MRI ordered, which was a terrifying thought, if only because it was becoming increasingly evident that whatever was wrong might lie in my skull.

Two weeks after my initial consultations, and plenty of sleepless nights later, I made my way to the local medical imaging lab for my very first MRI of what would be many to follow. My fear was intense—not so much over the MRI machine, but over what they might find. As a courtesy to my sanity, the friendly tech handed me a list of music options that I could choose to listen to while in the MRI tube. She told me to go ahead and write down the number corresponding to my selection. After selecting the Beatles Anthology on the music list, I slipped the supplied headphones over my head and nervously laid on the MRI table, trying to keep an open mind at what the results would be. After thirty minutes of buzzing, whirring, beeping and bleeping, one of the techs slid me out and said something she really shouldn't have said. "We need to take a few more slides. We're seeing something pretty big on your pituitary." What the hell did that mean? If there is one thing my medical experiences have taught me is to have an enormous respect for all levels of medical workers. Most of these people can be nothing short of angels at your side, but in this particular instance, I can't think of a more thoughtless thing anyone has ever said to me. A little candy coating wouldn't have hurt here, could it have? The next thirty minutes of my life seemed interminable in the MRI machine, as my imagination worked at a terrifying pace. After another 30 heart pounding minutes, I was pulled from the machine and was asked to stand up. I was finished. The experience here was worsened when I inquired about what had been seen. Another tech quickly snapped "That's not fair to us; you'll get results when you see your doctor!" I'm grateful that such people as these have dedicated their lives to administering these tests and that our technological advancements have come so far that machines can peer into the centers of our heads without so much as a pinch, but this was an inhuman way to handle someone who was just told they had "seen something pretty big" while doing medical scans of his head. Nevertheless, it was evident that the worker who had made the quick retort wasn't interested in negotiating. I remember the drive back to my apartment for the day, too shocked to cry and very thirsty but too depressed to stop for a drink. "What do I tell my fiancée, my parents, my friends?" I thought. Then the rational voice in my head would kick in and I'd think, "But you really don't know what's wrong, if anything. Stop it!" The only thing that got me through this stage was that rational voice always trying to climb over the fearful one. It was all hanging in the air with no concrete answers at that point.

The following few days were some of the most nerve-wracking days of my life. I told my experiences in the MRI to my fiancée, who immediately took in the same shock as I had. I'm having vision problems. We knew that. We knew something was on those slides taken in the MRI. Beyond that, we were limited in knowledge, so we did our best to not talk or worry about it. Despite our effort to quell any conversation, I did a pretty good job of hiding my irrational obsession with finding an answer. I had performed internet searches galore on all things intracranial. One word of advice for anyone with any pending diagnosis is to not, under any circumstances, browse the internet before you know the final results and full extent of your own individual case. I made this mistake and paid dearly for it with even more anxiety—as if I wasn't up to my ears in it already. I would personally recommend holding off on research until a diagnosis has been made. Once you know what you have, then it becomes critical that you know enough about it to communicate effectively with your doctor on treatment and symptoms.

Not long after the MRI, I found myself back in my neurologist's office with my loving fiancée at my side. As the door swung open, I thought, "This is it." I shared a quick glance of worried excitement with my fiancée and then shifted my eyes toward the stoic look on the doctor's face. At best, I'll be walking out of here today planning a celebration, and at worst…well, let's not go there. My neurologist looked at me and, asked "How do you feel?" I said "I feel ok," which was a lie, as my heart was in my throat. He immediately slid the MRI films into the light box and with no hesitation proclaimed, "You've got a tumor on your pituitary!" This was a mixed feeling, I remember. On one hand, I was terrified, but there was a glimmer of hope on the other hand. My endless internet searches yielded enough to inform me that pituitary tumors (also known as pituitary adenomas) were relatively common, often treatable, and most importantly almost always benign. I was relieved by the cold comfort that it most likely was not cancerous; but not all that relieved because there was, well…a tumor in the middle of my head. And it was large. The adenoma was so large in fact, that it received the coveted "giant macroadenoma" status – which really means nothing, other than a confirmation that it's a big one. The films revealed a 5 cm x 4 cm x 3.5 cm mass, which had grown itself around both carotid arteries and invaded many of the surrounding structures. The tumor had grown large enough to pressure my optic nerves, thus causing my vision problems. Little did I know at the time that this was only half of the diagnosis.

After my doctor shared the MRI results with me, I was referred to an endocrinologist for blood work to see what, if any, hormones were affected or being secreted. So I was on to see another specialist. When the endocrinologist walked in, he started his initial consultation with a whole host of strange questions involving my appearance, mental state. and just about everything else I could imagine. While possibly a little embarrassed, I felt that my endocrinologist knew what he was dealing with but would not specify anything because only blood work could confirm this diagnosis. And confirm it, it did. I was somewhat skeptical of the results, maybe even in denial when I went to have my initial labs done. I knew of the changes I felt were caused by excessive growth hormone, and things such as my underbite and swollen hands were more than a red flag, but I still held out hope. This hope was shattered when a week after my blood draw, I learned that my growth hormone (GH) and insulin-like growth factor (IGF-1) were at grossly elevated levels for a person of my age and sex. Further tests revealed abnormally low cortisol, testosterone, thyroid, and several other important hormones. These deficiencies were at the root of my mood and energy symptoms. I left my doctor's office that day a diagnosed acromegalic. "What an ugly word," I thought. "Of all things in this world, I get this obscure, rare, and strange disease!" I was happy on one hand that, while rare, this disease is quite treatable and well-researched. On the other hand, I was depressed and anxious at the road that lay ahead. It was a mixed bag of emotions, and I'll even admit that I had found some shred of humor in all of it. "Just my luck!" I thought, and I even took a bit of an "I'm special" attitude, much the same way a kid may show up to class one day with a cast and tell the story for show-and-tell.

The first step in combating this disease for me was surgery. I was fortunate in that my fiancée's father is an orthopedic surgeon, who was good friends with an experienced pituitary surgeon. While I did have two other consults, I decided to go with my fiancée's father's friend, as I felt most comfortable with him. I wasn't happy to have to have this type of surgery, but after reading accounts of patients who had pituitary surgery, I was comforted in knowing that as far as intracranial surgeries go, there are scarier procedures.

Shortly after my surgery was scheduled for October of 2006, life in our family would become even more stressful. Since my fiancée was at work and could not attend, my mother offered to drive me to the pre-operative appointment, which was a generous offer since the hospital was about an hour's drive away. She was concerned over my vision and how it would affect my ability to drive. I took the half-day off of work, and drove the short distance from my apartment to my parents' home. When I arrived, I walked in to my mother conversing on the phone. Normally, I wouldn't mind, but we were already running late, and I kept trying to pressure her to get off the phone so we could make my appointment. Frustrated, I told her I would be waiting in the car for her when she was done. Roughly ten minutes later, she emerged from her home and we were on our way. She asked how I felt, and, as I normally do, I said, "I feel okay." Mom's reply was nothing I would have even thought was possible. "Well, I just received some bad medical news myself." she said. The tone in her voice made it evident that she had more than the flu. She informed me she was on the phone with her doctor and had just received a diagnosis of stage III colorectal cancer. After I was diagnosed, I didn't think that things could have gotten any worse, but I was painfully wrong. This news was emotionally catastrophic, as it was following in the wake of my own medical crisis. After a great deal of conversation, which ranged from "why us" sulking to "let's fight this together" encouragement, I brought it up that our roads to recovery may have a similar treatment path. I knew enough about cancer treatment that it usually first involved chemotherapy, then a combination of surgery and radiotherapy. I mentioned to her that radiation was a possibility for my condition depending on the surgical outcome. In fact, I was told that because of the size of my tumor, radiation was a strong possibility.

Two weeks after mom shared her own medical challenges with me, my surgery was underway; and happily, things went well. Due to the fact that the hospital was very busy, I was confined to intensive care for 48 hours of the three and a half days I was to spend in the hospital. While the experience was certainly no fun, the surgery was relatively painless overall, considering I had someone poking around in my head. I was tended to by a caring staff of nurses and other medical professionals. My fiancée spent the first full day at my side as I was stuck in intensive care, due to the individual rooms being overpopulated. She's a brave soul for this, as screams of pain from surrounding partitions were the norm and our main form of entertainment was a television with no sound. We didn't speak much, as I was put on heavy pain killers and received an occasional dose of morphine. I was eventually moved to my own room after a miserable 48 hours in intensive care. This was a big upgrade! I had my own room in a newly built state-of-the-art wing of the hospital. I had a DVD player at my disposal, and my fiancée was allowed to sleep the night on a bed next to mine. I don't know how I would have gotten through this without my fiancée. Again, not always up for conversation, she gladly cycled DVDs in and out, and she held my hand when blood draws were taken and when—gasp—the nasal packing was removed. She even held the IV drip as I was given the green light to leave the room for a walk. I spent only one full day in this room. On the way home we stopped for pizza. Surgery was done!

A day later, my surgeon phoned me and enthusiastically told me that he had managed to pull a significant amount of the tumor out. This was the first good news I had received in a long while. Shortly after, my mom began her first rounds of chemotherapy. Shortly after this, a follow-up MRI was scheduled, as well as more blood tests. Unfortunately, my MRI revealed significant tumor remnants—mostly what had grown into structures deemed inoperable. Blood work also revealed still-elevated growth hormone levels, albeit reduced from pre-surgical numbers. Even though my levels weren't ideal, I did take note of a very sharp decrease in my facial and hand swelling. Over the course of a month or so, I began to see my cheek bones pointing out as they once did, and my fingers began losing their sausage-like appearance. It should also be noted here that my vision completely returned to normal within two weeks after surgery, thanks to the surgeon removing enough of the mass to relieve the pressure being exerted onto my optic nerves. While some tumor remained, I considered it a success in that symptoms were significantly relieved – something that gave me hope and more happiness than I had seen in a long time.

Since GH and IGF-1 levels were still elevated to an "unsafe" zone, more aggressive medical therapy was the next logical step to take in combating this disease. My endocrinologist put me on the middle dose of a monthly shot that is generally seen as the current gold-standard of Acromegaly medical therapies. But after three months on it, my blood work revealed zero change. I was disappointed, but options still remained and I was put on the highest dose of the drug, plus a dopamine. After three more months of this dosage and combination, guess what? Zero change. I was one of the not-so-lucky twenty percent or so of people who do not respond to this therapy. At this point I began to get very nervous about my options in fighting this disease. I was aware that the next step may involve radiotherapy if I opted for it. Despite this setback and the heavy decision it would be to undergo radiation, my fiancée and I remained resilient. We were certainly nervous, but we had seen through this battle enough to know that hope still existed.

There are two reasons why doctors who specialize in Acromegaly find radiation therapy an effective treatment. First, it's been shown to gradually decrease the prime cause of Acromegaly, the overproduction of growth hormone, although it can take years, and even decades to normalize such levels. The other benefit of radiation is that in a majority of cases, further growth of the tumor was either halted or partially reversed. Despite these benefits, there are significant drawbacks to such treatment. Anybody opting for radiotherapy to treat their Acromegaly shouldn't take the option lightly. There is a near one hundred percent incidence of further hypopituitarism (the *under*production of pituitary hormones) following radiation treatment. Also, there is a small but significant chance of a second tumor developing, tumors that can be *cancerous*! Other side effects are temporary, but no less painful for the patient dealing with them: effects include hair loss, skin irritation and fatigue. If you are concerned about sterility, I would strongly suggest you speak to your doctor about this before opting for radiotherapy.

Because of the previously mentioned drawbacks, radiation wasn't something I felt very comfortable about, and the decision weighed heavily. After my initial consult with a radiologist, and second, then third opinions, I hesitantly arrived at the conclusion that I would have to undergo this treatment. My fiancée had accompanied me to most of my consults, which afforded me a great deal of confidence that I was making the right decision. My fiancée and I were terrified of further tumor growth, which would almost certainly affect my vision again, and the remaining tumor was producing enough GH to continue to cause irreversible damage with its onslaught of ever-present symptoms. Another factor affecting my decision was the fact that first-line medical therapy was showing little, if any, effect, so my options were limited. Even though I was looking better due to the small decrease in GH post-surgery, my blood pressure was still high, and I was pre-diabetic, which has its own set of symptoms that usually involved a significant amount of fatigue at certain times of the day.

There are two main types of radiation used to treat acromegalic patients. These are stereotactic and conventional. Stereotactic radiosurgery is a newer approach, which allows a patient to receive a single large dose of radiation in one treatment session. Conventional radiation is a series of smaller doses of radiation delivered over the course of several weeks. My first choice was to seek consult for stereotactic radiosurgery because of the single-dose convenience, the increased efficacy over conventional radiation, and the fact that some studies showed lowered incidence of additional complications, including hypopituitarism. Unfortunately, I was not a candidate for radiosurgery. The tumor was too close in proximity to my optic nerves. This would make a single large dose of radiation an extreme danger to my vision. The only option in my case was a six-week course of conventional radiation. This procedure delivers many lower-dose beams that optic nerves and other important structures can withstand.

The first step in preparing for radiation treatment is a very thorough imaging process. This is done with, you guessed it, another MRI. I was getting quite used to the buzzing and blipping of those machines. I have a habit of falling asleep mid-scan and consider myself a very lucky person in regards to my lack of claustrophobia. I feel for the people who must undergo this who don't like the confinement. Current technology allows for the doctors to conform the series of beams to the exact volume of your tumor—a technique known as 3D conformal radiotherapy. More specifically, I was to undergo a version of 3D conformal therapy known as Intensity Modulated Radiation Therapy (IMRT), which not only allows the beams to be fired to the exact volume of my tumor, but each beam is set to its own level of intensity in regards to where the beam was being fired. This process allows the beams hitting the tumor to remain intense, and beams passing healthy tissue to be less intense, thus reducing damage to normal tissue. Some silver lining in all of this is that I learned a tremendous amount of what is out there in terms of medical procedures. Learning how nuanced and well-researched all of this was gave me a great deal of faith, and in many ways I found it very interesting.

The information gathered from the initial targeting MRI is entered into a computerized treatment planning system (TPS). This is a software system which allows the physicians to outline the tumor and then generate data to be used by physicians to devise an optimal treatment plan. When my Radiation Oncologist had what he believed to be the best course of action, I was called in to undergo a simulation. This simulation is used to double-check the treatment plan, and it is an introduction to what each day's treatment will be like. This is also the time at which you will have a custom face mask created. This is done by stretching a heated mesh template over your face and fastened to the table behind your head. The mesh template is then removed and heated, which hardens and fixes the mask in place. The mask is used to position your head in the exact position for each treatment day. This was one of the more bizarre aspects of radiation treatment. There is an unsettling feeling about having my head pinned to a table, and seeing my own face staring back at me as a lifeless sculpture of mesh was a reality-check for me. It set in to me that I was about to undergo six weeks of radiotherapy—a year earlier this was unfathomable. Fortunately for me, many of these initial negative feelings went away after the initial shock. The reassurances from the medical staff at the oncology facility were also a big help in alleviating concerns. Raising questions is a good thing. What are the side effects? How severe will they become? Does this treatment affect other systems in my body? How long can we expect to see results? Remember, no question is a dumb question. This disease is serious and so is your journey to remain healthy and happy. It's a good point to remember that every center has a counselor available to speak with when things get overwhelming.

I had an appointment afterwards with my physician, in which he spent a great deal of time with me going over each step of the process, what to expect, and when. I was given special head cream to be rubbed on each morning. This cream was to lessen the skin irritation effects, if I had any. He explained that hair loss was common, but luckily, with this type of radiation, the loss is spotty and in some people is virtually unnoticeable. I can see hair loss being a huge factor in deciding on radiation, but fear not, if I am any gauge, it grows back rather quickly after treatment. Fatigue is also a very big concern, and something that had me worried because as most people with Acromegaly know, energy levels are usually already compromised. Fortunately, I was told that the fatigue is late-onset and is rarely severe. This consult was nicely reassuring, and I felt a bit more enthusiastic about getting back at that damned tumor—this time we'll fry it!

Several days later, I received a phone call from the Radiation Oncologist informing me that everything looked as it should and we were ready to start our schedule. My treatment plan would involve daily treatments for six weeks, excluding weekends; and I was to have 10 points of radiation delivery per session. My employer was very understanding and allowed me to leave 2 hours early each day for the duration of treatment. I had a record with my current employer as being someone who goes beyond the call of duty, and of working fast and efficiently. I was fortunate that I worked for someone who recognized this. I began treatment on a Monday, and I was very nervous, but that seemed natural. My fiancée, as she always did, went out of her way to accompany me and to show her support. This worked out for her most days because she worked in the area, and the days when she worked her early shift, she was able to leave by 3:00 p.m., whereas my daily treatment was between 4:00 p.m. and 5:00 p.m. Despite the convenience, there's no doubt this routine must have been exhausting for her, as I know it was for me.

To tell the truth, the second I sat down in the waiting room, all of the fear, terror, anxiety and depression came roaring back, and everything seemed "too real" again. My fiancée and I took two of the few available seats in the waiting room after we signed in. To my left was a table with a half-completed jigsaw puzzle, which an elderly man was patiently piecing together. To our right, a middle-aged woman sat with her head down and half-asleep. In front of us was another man, no older than 40, sitting in a wheelchair and receiving oxygen from a tank; I assumed it was his mother who sat next to him and seemed to be giving him comforting words. Behind us and to the right were the two treatment rooms, sealed off by large metal doors to prevent radiation overflow. Adjacent to the treatment rooms was another room where the tech's punched buttons and administered treatment. There were many more people, almost all dressed in aprons and awaiting their treatments. And there was me, sitting among them. Out of respect, I tried desperately not to guess at what had been their diagnosis and what their journey to this room must have been like. This also brought me back to thoughts of my mom, as she recently sat in another room very similar to this. I hated the thought that anybody in my family or any stranger in this room had to go through this misery. Strangely, I actually felt guilty. For all my grief and heartache over my diagnosis, I imagine there were far worse things in this room, and my perspective shifted a little bit. I picked up an outdated People magazine and pretended to read. This is where I was to spend afternoons for the next month and a half.

I spent forty anxious minutes or so waiting, when one of the techs emerged from the back and called my name. I had a brief burst of nervous adrenaline, stood up and kissed my fiancée. "Good luck!" she said. The tech was friendly and attentive, as they always were at the treatment center. She escorted me to the treatment room and gestured to head inside. Through a thick metal sliding door, a lone table sat in the center of a gray, lifeless room. Above the table and behind sat the linear accelerator – the actual machine that delivers the doses of radiation. I was asked to lie on the table, lay my head onto the headrest, and adjust myself into a comfortable position. The staff took great effort to assure my comfort, asking me if I would like a blanket or if I had questions. I felt as comfortable as I could, refused a blanket and stated that I was ready for my first treatment. They carefully placed my mask over my face and snapped it into the fastening below. The staff left the room and closed and sealed the door behind them. I was still quite nervous, but I assured myself that I was making the right decision.

A minute after the staff had left the room, a voice came over the loudspeaker informing me that treatment was about to begin and asked one last time if I was comfortable. "Yes," I said. "Okay, the piece of equipment above your head will begin to move; try to stay still," the voice said. The machine began a slow, smooth motion to the right of my head, which was to be the first of ten positions, or ports, that summed up each treatment session. Once the machine was in position, it seemed to make a few micro-adjustments, stop, adjust a bit more, stop, and then buzz. The buzzing was when the machine was administering the radiation, and it lasted about twenty seconds. Still nervous, this very first step in treatment relieved a lot of tension. It was painless, and my head didn't explode like it had in my "worst-case scenario" scenario. No more than ten seconds after the first buzzing, the machine had shifted a bit into the second position. This buzz lasted slightly longer than the first dose. This second dose I imagined had a clearer shot at the tumor, thus it lasted a tad longer. About this time, I tried to make the best of the current circumstances, and I began to personify my tumor. I imagined it as this little hell raising demon, finally getting what it deserved. After surgery, this was round two, and he wasn't getting away this time! It wasn't much, but this idea was amusing enough to get my mind off of the reality of the situation. Throughout the session, the machine made its way around my head from right to left, stopping at each of the ten points of entry along the way. The whole process had me on the table for about half an hour. As soon as I counted the tenth dose, it was no more than a minute before the door opened and the tech unlatched my mask from the clips. "You're done for the day!" he said. "How was it?" "Not too bad," I replied. I thanked him and I was on my way home for the day.

Each daily treatment was essentially unremarkable. However, one thing to note, and a very odd thing, is that when the machine positioned itself nearer my right temple and began the dose in the third position, I noticed of a very strange metallic, bleach-like smell. About the fifth or sixth treatment I inquired about this and learned that in some people, the radiation passing through the brain can create an olfactory response, thus you "smell" the radiation. I was told that others see lights. When I was assured this didn't mean anything dangerous, I found it kind of amusing.

The six weeks, which seemed daunting at first, actually moved rather quickly. Before I knew it, I was three weeks into treatment—half way home! Outside of my daily afternoon treatment sessions, things were pretty much normal. I worked 7:30 a.m. to 3 p.m. every day, drove an hour to treatment, sat in treatment about an hour, and was always the last person out of treatment. This was a good thing, as much of the staff was getting ready to head home and were more talkative with me than other patients since their work was done. There were certainly good days and bad days. Bad days were the days in which my fiancée worked an early shift, which she did three days a week, and would be out the door for work before I was awake. By the end of the day, I would get home around 6:30, and she would be asleep on the couch. We didn't see each other all that often. Although we lived in a cramped apartment, our surrounding area was nice, and we had made a habit of walking to a local lake several days out of the week from the time we moved in. We did that after work usually, and it was always a nice way to end the day and to allow us to forget our stressors. During treatment, we were not able to find the time to do this, and even such a small thing only added to the heartache of it all. Weekends were our salvation. We never planned much other than sitting around our apartment or visiting my parents and taking their dog for a walk. We didn't want to plan much during this time, as the weekdays were often too much, and doing nothing on the weekends was as much bliss as we could have asked for. But all this was manageable knowing I would be done with treatments within a few weeks. I did also feel a bit fatigued, but nothing that hindered work. I simply had to take it a bit easier than usual. I also had a moderate amount of hair loss, which was a series of quarter-sized patches which matched the positioning of the ten daily doses. This too wasn't a problem for me because it was hardly noticeable. I continued to rub the cream on my scalp each day, which resulted in a very odd rash. When I brought this up to my doctor, he switched me to the "unscented" cream, because a few people react this way. My fiancée and I laughed hysterically at this revelation that I was using the scented version, as we both had joked at how awful the stuff had smelled.

By the end of the six-week cycle, I was completely unphazed by the hour-long commute, even though I was suffering a mild amount of exhaustion. I was very much ready to end this treatment and hope for the best. My very last treatment was as routine as the others. However, I was delighted to find the small staff of technicians who had overseen my treatment standing all together when I exited the treatment room for the last time. I got a round of applause, a few congratulatory words and a farewell. Best of all I got a "certificate of completion" which now hangs on my office wall as an amusing reminder of my trials with Acromegaly. Sure, a certificate is silly, but it's little things like that which can take the edge off. I thanked them for all of their hard work and left the building for the last time. They also let me keep the face mask, which I've appropriately spray-painted black and now have hanging in my garage as another reminder of all I've had to endure.

My radiation treatment started and ended three years ago. Several months after my treatments ended, I went in for a follow-up MRI and received the results that the tumor had actually shrunk by about twenty percent. This was great news! While the tumor still lies close to my optic chiasm, it's been stable with no further signs of growth. Serum GH concentrations also fell a bit following radiation and subsequently so did IGF-1 levels. I still have elevated GH levels when off medication, but radiation did reduce my levels. The good news is that there has been a steady decrease in serum GH over the past three years following oral glucose testing. It's not unreasonable to believe that I will reach normal levels without medication sometime in the near future. I still take a daily shot, and take thyroid and testosterone replacements. I am happy to say that I am, as far as I'm concerned, symptom-free when it comes to swelling, growth, headaches and all the routine complications. Unfortunately, I did lose my ability to have children of my own, but I don't let that get me down as I know there are some things that can be done for this, and adoption is certainly an option. I continue to receive annual MRIs, and have routine blood work every six months. Many days go by when I simply don't even think about the fact that I have such a disease. My now-wife and I have since found new work and bought our first home. I have more energy today than I ever have had in my entire life. I have even taken up participating in triathlons as my new hobby. My mom continues her cancer treatments, and is, at the time of this writing, in a second round of chemotherapy. We are, however, optimistic and expect a full remission.

If there is one thing I'd like to tell anyone diagnosed or with a loved one who has been diagnosed with Acromegaly, it is that I know from my own story and from many others I've spoken to over the years that you should expect better days. My initial days with this disease were extremely dark, but knowing what I do now, I can honestly sit back and reassure myself that I have long since made it into the light at the end of the tunnel.

Tyson Koerper was diagnosed with Acromegaly in 2006. He's currently in remission, and spends most of his time earning a living as a freelance graphic designer. In his spare time, he enjoys running, cycling, and training his two Siberian Huskies with his supportive wife, Aneil.

Dealing with the Disease: Friends and Family

Haley Zelenka

You sometimes need help navigating through that process. And this way, when you call, you're calling a person rather than just asking if there's somebody who can help you.

—Chip Cherry

The term "navigation" is the perfect articulation of my journey over the past nine years. While I have ventured down a variety of paths, experiencing struggles and success, and making lots of mistakes in the process, I have learned more about myself than I could have ever imagined. I never really thought of myself as the navigator of my own life until I sat down to reflect upon my journey and to share my experiences in dealing with Acromegaly, or more appropriately, to share my experiences in "navigating" through my journey with Acromegaly. I guess that I have always associated such a role with strength, tenacity, and autonomy, all qualities which I have never really exuded. However, in doing so, I seem to have forgotten that keeping a ship on its course requires more than an individual to direct its path. Even the navigator cannot manage the ship alone.

I think that I had always assumed, like the majority of other eighteen-year-olds, that leaving for college would be one of the most exciting, memorable times of my life. I remember distinctly the day that I sat in my third-floor dorm room watching my family drive away, tears steadily rolling down my cheeks. I'll never forget my mom whispering in my ear, "You don't have to do this," as she smiled and hugged me goodbye. I knew that I had to do it, but just hearing those words meant so much to me. As I sat there on the floor of my new home, I couldn't help but reflect upon the preceding months, and I decided at that moment that I had to do it. I had to achieve the goals which I had set for myself as a young child, to be something more than what I had become the past few months, and I made a commitment with myself to do it all on my own. Only a little over three months prior to that day, I had been diagnosed with a condition that I was struggling to understand, and a condition that I was sure nobody else would.

I can describe my childhood and adolescence as nothing less than fantastic. I was constantly surrounded by people who loved me, and I was reminded of that love daily. Growing up, I was content spending time at home with my brother and sister, and some of my fondest memories include trips to the Aquatic Club and great meals at "The Dump" (when my brother and sister and I played restaurant, that was our restaurant's name). Having my extended family nearby was great too. I enjoyed spending time at my grandparents' home and looked forward to holiday gatherings. My parents dedicated every ounce of themselves to me and my younger brother and sister, and I was given more opportunities than I could have ever imagined. I prided myself in school involvement, and I participated in an array of extracurricular activities, never finding it difficult to make friends. I had, and arguably still have, all of the "oldest child" qualities, thus living primarily to make everyone else happy and gaining my own happiness in the process. Life was relatively easy, and I was content. I lived comfortably in my own perfect bubble and was not at all prepared for the inconveniences that resulted when I realized for myself that perfection just doesn't exist.

It was on April 16, 2002, that the ideal life to which I had grown so accustomed changed quite a bit. I had proceeded through the usual weekday routine, attempting eagerly to pass the time until I would be a high school graduate and enjoy the freedom and excitement associated with beginning life on my own. I had struggled through the first half of the school day with a drooping eyelid, and as the day progressed and no relief occurred, I visited the pediatrician that afternoon. Upon examination, I was written a prescription for an antibiotic cream intended to treat a likely sinus infection. The pediatrician who saw me that day seemed a little worried and, to be cautious, sent me for a CT scan. At that point, I don't know if it was the result of my own naiveté or the feeling that I was invincible, but I wasn't afraid. In fact, as guilty as I feel admitting it, when we arrived at the hospital shortly thereafter, I remember feeling happy for a welcome break from afternoon classes. In the midst of my own ignorance, I failed to notice the worry and concern which I know that my mother must have been feeling.

Not even the haste with which I was scheduled for testing, or the promptness in admitting me to the area for examination, caused me any apprehension. As far as I was concerned, I was at the hospital solely to undergo the precautionary testing which had been suggested by the doctor, and I complied willingly with the instructions of the technicians. As a dedicated *ER* fan, I recognized some of the large medical devices that I had seen on television, and I remember being somewhat fascinated with the idea of getting a firsthand glimpse at their operation. Things become a little blurry after I emerged slowly from underneath the machine which had blatantly portrayed the unexpected mass that appeared on my brain. I remember being placed in a tunnel-like MRI machine, with which I would later become very familiar. After what felt like an eternity, as I lay there wondering what was wrong with me and whether or not I was going to die, I was pulled out and greeted by a few concerned looks and what looked like stray tears on my mom's cheek. It was at that moment that I knew my drooping eyelid was a little more serious than a sinus infection.

Without receiving much explanation from the physicians who had performed the tests and made such serious observations, I was placed in a hospital room where I remained for several days. I remember finally asking the doctors directly what was wrong with me, and the information that I received initially was an illustration sketched on the marker board in the hospital room. Seeing the rough depiction of my brain and the tumor affixed thereto made it real, and I looked up at the board many times. Tests continued, and each day my fears became a little more intense. In the process of surveying the tumor, described by one doctor as the size of a child's fist, the pieces of this mysterious puzzle began to fall into place. I distinctly remember the visual field test and the apprehension that I experienced as I sat there unable to see the blinking dots. Unbeknownst to me, as a result of the pressure of the tumor against my optic nerve, I had lost all vision in my left eye; and surprisingly, at that time my vision seemed like the least of our worries. Surgery was scheduled immediately, and it wasn't long before the news of a brain tumor literally made the papers. As can be imagined, such a story was certainly a rarity in a small town on the coast of Mississippi; but the outreach was anything but rare. The support that I received during that time was overwhelming. I was never alone in that hospital room, and I never had any doubt that I was loved. Even with all of the support and love, however, I don't think that I have ever been more scared in my life. I had no idea what was happening to me.

Surgery was scary, but I had no hesitation in entrusting myself to a gifted and caring surgeon who recognized my fears. While the procedure resulted in only partial removal of the tumor, due primarily to the proximity of the tumor to the optic nerve, it was certainly successful. Almost immediately, I regained nearly all of the vision that I had lost, and that was reassuring news. The days following were painful, but the relief associated with the word *benign* made the discomfort a lot easier to endure. Not long after recovery, I began the plodding and disheartening quest for answers. For me, the road seemed so long and difficult. While I can't recall any initial discussion, the word *Acromegaly* had been mentioned during my time in the hospital, specifically after the initial blood tests showed elevated IGF-1 levels. Several weeks later, I got the "official" diagnosis from an endocrinologist and began medical therapy shortly thereafter. During the first few months, it seemed as though my parents and I met quite a few endocrinologists before we actually received a thorough explanation of the disease. Maybe it was just the result of my being eighteen and much more concerned with the other aspects of life at the time, but I don't remember ever sitting down with a doctor and obtaining any kind of understanding. While the diagnosis was certainly overwhelming, it was also a little comforting. The unusual changes in my body and the frequent visits to the pediatrician over the past few years made a little more sense, and it became frighteningly obvious just how different I looked from the other members of my immediate family.

Prior to my diagnosis, I had never had any serious health problems aside from an occasional running injury and a minor cold, and I was frequently teased by my family for my obnoxiously healthy eating habits. In retrospect, though, the signs and symptoms had been present for years. As an avid runner and overall active young woman, I maintained a healthy lifestyle and a generally slim stature. Looking back, however, I had experienced noticeable weight gain over the span of just a few years and couldn't attribute it to any change in my lifestyle, even despite a physician's recommendation that I simply needed to "push away from the table." Additionally, I had several instances of swelling in my hands and feet, and I distinctly remember stepping off the plane after a family trip to Hawaii and not being able to fit my swollen feet back into my shoes. Around that same time, I had become extremely self-conscious of the intense sweating that was beginning to occur quite frequently. As individual occurrences, the symptoms went easily unnoticed, but after diagnosis, the signs seemed so much more apparent.

Throughout the process of obtaining relief for a mysterious condition which we knew little about, I was prescribed a number of medications, all of which took a severe toll on my body and spirit. In addition to the physical changes that I had experienced from the years with Acromegaly, steroids and extreme dosages of various drugs made things even worse. I gained nearly sixty pounds within a few months and had still not received any real explanation concerning my condition and the result of the growth hormone–producing tumor that had engulfed my pituitary gland. Unlike most acromegalics who spend the majority of their lives experiencing debilitating symptoms, only to be diagnosed with the disease well into adulthood, my diagnosis occurred during a unique phase of my life. Whether it was naivety or fear, I ignored the reality of the situation for as long as I could, placing such a tremendous burden on my already-apprehensive parents. As embarrassing as it is to admit, my focus was not so much on the more serious risks of heart disease and diabetes. I was most concerned with my physical appearance and the inconvenience that the disease might have on my college plans.

Having been diagnosed with the disease at such an early age, I relied primarily upon my parents not only for support, but for guidance, advice, and most importantly, their determination to get only the best medical support available. As much as I hate to admit it, I passed along most responsibilities to my parents. I let them worry, and I let them ask the important questions. My mom spent endless hours researching the disease online, and there is no doubt that she was more versed on the subject than I could have ever imagined being. She brought along her black notebook to each doctor visit, and she knew exactly which questions to ask. My dad always listened so intently to the doctors, but he was also always there to listen to me as well, helping me calm my fears and reminding me that I made him "so proud his heart hurt," words written in a card that I will cherish forever. I think I always knew that I was so lucky to have such a zealous pair behind me, but I also know that I took that for granted. Typical of a child, I liked the attention that I received as a result of the situation, but I wasn't willing to take responsibility for my health. I was content passing on the difficult tasks, and my parents so willingly embraced them.

Unfortunately, in spite of my parents' best efforts, not every medical experience was ideal. While discouraging words and blatant apathy may have gone easily overlooked by a child like myself, my parents had no problem demanding accountability and compassion. In our lengthy quest for answers, or at least a little understanding, we met a few doctors who were more than willing to discount our concerns and to minimize my mysterious symptoms without even knowing me. I was much more than just another patient to my parents, and they sought to shield me not only from the disease itself but also from the slightest indication of negativity. Even now, at twenty-seven years old and some nine years since diagnosis, I still notice my parents' inherent need to protect me, and I know there are things that they will never share with me about that period of my life. I'm okay with that, though. For me, it was imperative that I adjust to this new stage from my own perspective and observations.

It's really fascinating, especially after hearing stories now about that time in 2002, that my memory is based solely upon my recollection of the experience as a high school senior. While I commenced this medical expedition with lots of others, I also underwent a journey of my own. I attempted to make sense of the information that I had absorbed from doctors, drug reps, and even Internet searches. I spent lots of time lying in bed thinking about it all. During that time, not only did I begin to appreciate the disease, the symptoms, the results, and the changes, but I also began to appreciate myself and the experiences that I knew were yet to come.

Once I recovered fully from surgery and once we had all digested the initial shock of diagnosis, we began the overwhelming process of surveying treatment options and determining the best route for me. Due to such elevated IGF-1 levels, it was imperative that I begin medical therapy as quickly as possible, which ended up being about two months after surgery. Still, though, there were long-term decisions regarding treatment that had to be made. Hearing the word *radiation* was frightening enough, and with the array of pharmaceutics which had been mentioned by a number of healthcare individuals, my feelings of hopelessness were only exacerbated. I had embarked upon a steady emotional decline, and I turned primarily to isolation and denial. I just knew that my plans for college were over, or at least significantly delayed, and at eighteen, that thought was the worst of them all. Putting aside my selfishness and immaturity, however, I did sit down with my parents and physician to discuss the ongoing effects of medical therapy. Not only was it all foreign to me and to my parents, these treatments were also new to the medical field as a whole, making our assessment even more difficult and seemingly much less "informed."

For me, medical therapy seemed most conducive to my lifestyle and appeared as though it would cause minimal interruption in my life. At that time, my options were limited, so deciding upon the type of medication wasn't at all difficult. I received little information about the drug prior to beginning therapy and felt as if I was embarking blindly upon this medical journey. As frightening as it sounds now, I relied solely upon the advice and suggestion of a physician who appeared equally as unfamiliar with the medication and also with the disease itself. I did realize almost immediately, however, that the medication intake would be quite different than any other medication which I had ingested previously. Adjusting to intramuscular (given by needle into the muscle) and subcutaneous (under the skin) administration would be particularly difficult, especially in light of the fact that I had no idea what either of those words meant. Without much demonstration, I received my first injection at the physician's office and was released to begin my own injection arrangements each month.

Sure, the needle was massive, I thought to myself, but a shot a month couldn't possibly be that difficult. Not to mention, that idea sounded like a perfect way to salvage the plans which I had spent so much of my life meticulously planning. At that point, I needed an escape, a place where I could redefine myself, a place where nobody knew about the past few months of my life. When I opted for continued medical therapy over radiation and/or more surgery, I also made the decision to attend college a few hours north of home, quite a convenient balance for starting anew while also ensuring that I could make it home once a month for the injection. Though I had little connection to Mississippi State University, I was drawn initially to the allure of entering a campus and leaving behind the worries, frustration, and the sadness that had consumed my final days in high school and the months preceding my freshman year of college. For the first time in a while, I had regained my sense of hope and determination, and I was motivated solely by a desire to rediscover the person that I had been only a few months before.

Preparing for the big move, I decided that I couldn't allow my disease to define me, and I was intent on keeping that part of my life separate from the new college life upon which I was embarking. I was fairly confident that any mention of a brain tumor would certainly send any potential new friends running in the opposite direction, and I hoped to be recognized as much more than a girl with some weird disease. As I discovered in the first few days, it was all much tougher than I had originally anticipated. The physical changes that I had experienced, combined with the symptoms of Acromegaly and the recent effects of a variety of medications, were the most difficult to overcome. In a matter of a few short months, I felt as if I had been transformed, through no fault of my own, from the happy, healthy young woman I had always been to an overweight, unattractive individual consumed with feelings of self-consciousness and embarrassment. I don't know why I believed that it was possible to leave those feelings behind, but it didn't take me long to find out that they were certainly not feelings that I could escape. It was a kind of unique inner conflict with which I struggled daily. On one hand, I wanted to shout my situation from the rooftops so that my peers wouldn't assume that I was lazy and repulsive. On the other hand, however, I wanted to keep that part of my life as far away from Starkville, Mississippi, as I could. I wanted to be a charmer; I wanted to fit in; I wanted to be a college student like everyone else, and I couldn't do that with a trail of excess growth hormone following behind me. Unfortunately, things weren't quite as easy as I had hoped. It didn't take long for my feelings of insecurity to completely consume me, and my extreme self-consciousness prevented me from interacting much with others.

As much as I wanted to ease my parents' worries and provide them with the assurance that I was well adjusted and happy, I inadvertently clung to them more than I realized. For a while, my communications with the outside world consisted solely of telephone conversations with family members—the ones that knew the old me, the me that was real, the me that was happy, and the me that was confident in the person that I once was. For the majority of my first semester, I let my Acromegaly completely control my life. I avoided social situations and spent lots of time alone feeling unworthy and insecure, making it much easier to hide my disease. I continued to obsess over the physical changes, and I made sure to work out at the gym early in the morning or late at night when I knew that it would be most empty. In an attempt to feel a little more confident in myself and my body, I would go days without eating, only to eventually find comfort in splurging on something unhealthy that I could get without having to see anyone. I traveled south once every month unnoticed and was able to spend that terrible "shot day" in the comfort of my home without having to offer anyone any explanation and without fearing that I would be deemed even more abnormal than I already was.

The second semester was a little less difficult. As I ventured outside of my comfort zone and sought contentment through campus involvement, I also managed to open myself up to some really special people—people who, without even knowing it, allowed me to begin rediscovering my own worth. With their acceptance, it became much easier to look past the insecurities which I had allowed to completely consume me and which had caused me to miss out on so many wonderful experiences. I slowly began the process of rediscovery, a process with which I continue to struggle some nine years later; and my willingness to share my medical situation with new friends confirmed my inherent need for understanding and support. Throughout my years in college and eventually in law school, I continued to rely on the same few special people in my life, people willing to accept me even when I had difficulty accepting myself.

While diagnosis and the initial quest for achieving a sense of relief and control were extremely challenging, the years following haven't always been easy either. Frequent doctor visits, MRIs, blood tests, daily and monthly injections, gall stones, and the occasional headache have been a few of the additional obstacles. Never anything more than I could handle. In the midst of it all, I've stumbled upon a pretty steady foundation. Throughout the years following diagnosis, opening myself up to others provided me with the little comforts of home, even when I was away from it. I never felt more special than when my friends willingly sacrificed a Friday night out on the town to stay in and watch movies with me, as I lay there recovering from the injection that I had received that afternoon. I even relished the jokes we would make about my situation because those jokes provided me with the assurance that I was accepted and loved unconditionally. To this day, I can't help but smile when I think of the endearing title "Yabadabadoo feet," knowing that it represents a comforting approval of the real me, even with my not-so-attractive, large feet, and even now, nothing tastes better than "tumor juice."

During my own lengthy process of acceptance and the mistakes that I have made therein, I am fortunate enough to have learned one of the greatest lessons in life. While self-reliance is certainly an admirable quality, the unconditional support of others is truly a gift that cannot be surpassed. I attempted to battle my disease, and the unfortunate effects that resulted, solely on my own, and I lost a part of myself in the process. Unfortunately, it is when you can't seem to love yourself that you truly realize just how important the love and support of friends and family really is. Informing others of my past medical history and current struggles has become essentially a rite of passage, an indicator of my trust for the individual in whom I am confiding. Acknowledging my condition and the effects thereof forces me to emerge from the mask in which I hide from so many and to confront the person I am, albeit with imperfections. While the process is certainly liberating, it remains extremely difficult.

Acromegaly, like any other disease, is never consistent among those who suffer from it. No two patients will experience all of the same symptoms, the same emotions, the same treatment, or the same struggles. Nevertheless, it is most comforting to recognize a sense of camaraderie among the lucky few, even in the loneliest of times. I think it's natural to find support in those to whom you can relate, and it can be a little disheartening to feel like you don't have anyone. It's difficult to explain what not feeling right means. People want to help, but it's difficult to describe how someone else can help you when you don't really know how to help yourself. I am confident that every person diagnosed with Acromegaly, regardless of his or her age or lifestyle, has experienced that same feeling, and knowing that is much more powerful than any drug that we could ever be prescribed. I find myself frequently "diagnosing" strangers in my mind when I pass an individual and observe some of the seemingly distinctive Acromegaly symptoms and signs which we all know so well. While I certainly experience a feeling of compassion as I entertain such a thought, I can't help but smile knowing that a person also having suffered with Acromegaly firsthand, has made a similar recognition. It sounds crazy, and maybe it is, but it's an Acro thing that only a few special people could possibly understand.

Acromegaly, regardless of the strength of the individual diagnosed, is not a disease to tackle alone, and even with the strongest of support units, there will be difficult days. After nine years as an official "acromegalic," I still have those days when I feel alone and misunderstood. There are still days when I hide behind the disease and then criticize myself for yielding to self-pity and insecurity. There are still days when I regret allowing myself to submit to those feelings only to miss out on some really great experiences. My navigation is ongoing, and while some days are rougher than others, I have a pretty amazing crew to keep me going.

There is no doubt that my family and close friends have provided me with a support unit stronger than I could have ever imagined. Unfortunately, during the early months, I never spent much time considering the extent to which my condition and the inconveniences associated therewith had impacted those closest to me. Ever since I was a child, I have dreamed of being the big sister that my younger siblings would look up to, and as much as I still hope that I have made by brother and sister proud, I look up to them. I have learned so much about life by watching them endure the same experiences that I have, except with much more strength and resilience. Brain surgery and the frustrating months thereafter were certainly frightening for an eighteen-year-old, but the feelings that my family and friends were forced to endure certainly had to be much more difficult.

I have experienced a variety of emotions since diagnosis in 2002, but I have also come to better appreciate the relationships which I have formed over the years. I have discredited some pretty amazing people, and I have put myself and my own need for acceptance above them. I made it all about me, and I expected others to do the same. It was like I always thought that I had a free pass to treat others however I wanted and then blame my behavior on the disease. There were lots of times that, for whatever reason, I didn't like myself, and I made it easy for others not to like me either.

For me, Acromegaly has truly been a learning experience, a journey in which I plan to persist for the rest of my life. While Acromegaly will always be a part of who I am, I will refuse to allow it to define me, and I am confident that the same support which I have always received from my friends and family will allow me to continue to thrive as an individual, not simply an individual with a disease. I still find myself obtaining comfort with isolation, but it is interesting to see with whom I seek refuge when things are at their worst. To this day, I rely on those few people who I have been willing to welcome into my secret life. I still experience days of discouragement and hopelessness, but I am reminded constantly of just how blessed I am to have such a strong support system comprised solely of the people who love me most. I can only hope to provide that kind of support and encouragement to someone else.

There is no doubt that my family and friends have played such a significant role in helping me navigate my own journey. While I didn't realize it at the time of the experience, I now relish the memories that I've made over the past nine years and recognize the reasons that I dealt with situations and people the way that I did. I will never forget spending fun evenings with my cousins while my aunt, a registered nurse, waited on my medicine to reach room temperature. It didn't matter how bad the needle hurt going in, the pain never lasted long with my two-year-old cousin holding my hand the whole time and then asking if I was okay after everything was over. Just goes to show you, it's the little things that truly make it all bearable. A few years ago, I was lucky enough to stumble upon the endocrinologist who has changed my life simply by being himself and by treating me like an individual, not merely another patient. I have had an amazing opportunity to meet the special people who also share this disease, and I am so proud to be a part of this community. What a blessing these people have been in my life.

I don't want to make the misleading representation that I have overcome all of the painful aspects of Acromegaly. I simply have learned a little about management, about navigation, and about appreciating myself and those who have seen me through it all. To this day, I struggle constantly with nagging feelings of insecurity, anxiety, fear, and even hopelessness. I had a plan for my life, and it's difficult to accept the fact that things don't always go according to plan. I look around and compare myself frequently to the people around me, and then I worry that I have disappointed the people who love me. I question myself constantly, and I feel like I've remained stationary while everyone else is moving forward. As much as I hate to admit it, I find myself wishing sometimes that my life was a little simpler. But then again, if life were simple, it would be impossible for me to appreciate where I've been, what I've done, and how I've gotten there.

I like to think that I am becoming a better navigator each day. I have ventured down a variety of paths and made lots of mistakes in the process, and certainly will make many more, but I have learned to appreciate the role of my crew. I realize that the challenges will never recede completely, but I am reminded that I have the strength and support to manage my ship.

Haley Zelenka is a native of the Gulf Coast and is currently a practicing attorney in Gulfport, Mississippi. Haley graduated from Mississippi State University with a B.S. in English and went on to obtain her J.D. at the University of Mississippi. Committed to service, Haley devotes much of her practice to issues of family law, and she also possesses a strong passion for child advocacy and the protection of public interests and civil rights. Haley has acquired a similar passion for providing medical support, especially to those touched by Acromegaly, and she currently has the honor of serving on the Inaugural Board of Directors for Acromegaly Community. Inspired by her own journey with Acromegaly and the struggles associated therewith, Haley aspires to provide others with the support that she has so graciously received throughout her own experiences.

Dealing with Negativity in Your Life

Wayne Brown

Life is what happens to you while you're busy making other plans . . .

—John Lennon

Medical Issues Hit Me Early in Life

As a child, adults always said that Wayne doesn't know his size. While I did not really understand the sentiment, I heard that I was different from everyone else. I know that the adults were not trying to be malicious, but euphemisms can be very confusing to kids. When I heard that statement, I was usually playing, so I would pause to try to decipher what it meant; and I would go back to playing remembering that I was different. As an adult, I now understand that decoding subtext is a major life activity. As humans, not only do we have to manage our own lives and all its obstacles, we also have to fit within our community structure: family, friends, school, work, and total strangers. The big trick is to figure out how to make sure everybody you care about loves you as much as you love them, which is not always an easy feat when you are convinced that you are so different from the people in your community structure.

Everyone has heard the phrase that life is an adventure. Well, I am positive that few people have seen the amazing adventures I have enjoyed and endured. My life did not start out with all that much excitement or adventure . . . for at least the first few weeks! While I was born perfectly healthy with ten little fingers and ten little toes, that would not last for very long. My life's adventure started within a month of my birth, and it would be the love that my parents had for each other and their children that was most important, as we would lose countless hours at the local Children's Hospital. It's not that I was diagnosed with some exotic or unusual illness, but rather *when* I was diagnosed with a very common malady. I guess the upside is that I would have great preparation for later in life when I would again feel like the main exhibit at the local museum.

Before I was born, my thyroid did not grow where it was supposed to grow in my body, so the necessary hormones produced by the thyroid were unable to get to their specified body parts. Now, thyroid issues were already quite common by the 1970s, and synthetic thyroid had long been created, tested, and established in *adults.* At the time though, hypothyroidism was an adult problem. It's not that babies never had problems with their thyroids; it's just that a treatment protocol did not exist for infants *yet.* Suddenly there was an infant with a thyroid problem and a very strong-willed family. At the time of my birth, infants without an active thyroid had a ridiculously low survival rate, and those who did live were severely limited in their academic abilities. No surprise that after my problem was discovered, the doctors at the hospital gave me little-to-no chance to survive past infancy. Lucky for me that my pediatrician had recently read an article arguing that physicians should try using synthetic thyroid pills to treat infants and children with underproductive thyroids. Dr. Bobby, as I knew him, called my mom after he got the report from the hospital and said she needed to come in immediately. "And make sure you bring someone with you, besides the baby." Thankfully my mom was a new mom, so she did not stop to think that this meant bad news. She asked my grandfather (her father) to go with. Mom and papa went into the office only to hear the whole awful story unravel. After Dr. Bobby finished telling mom what was going on, he then asked right there whether she wanted to try the synthetic thyroid, knowing that the alternative was a likely death sentence. This is one of those medical "options" that does not really provide the patient with any reasonable options. Hmmm . . . do I want to take a long shot and let my baby be a human guinea pig, or do I just let my child die? I am very thankful that papa was there because she needed someone strong to keep her together. Our family network has always been solid, and my family rallied around my parents, willing to help with anything they needed.

Fast forward several months, my parents brought me to the hospital for one of my regular checkups to make sure I was growing normally, or at the very least to keep an eye on my progress for the articles that I would eventually inspire for who knows how many medical journals. It was on this day that my parents really learned the power that words hold. Some young doctor who was supposed to be a brilliant man had a brief lapse of genius when he told my parents that while it was good that I was responding to the medication and I was probably going to live, the likelihood was that my growth would be severely slowed, both mentally and physically. If I was lucky, the doctor said, I would only be mentally retarded, and quite possibly dependent on others for my life care. Needless to say, any parents would be absolutely beside themselves with grief, and my parents were first-time parents. They were absolutely destroyed… but equally defiant! Our family never took no for an answer from people in lab coats, and my parents were not going to start now. They made it their personal crusade to make sure I would be as able-bodied as could be realized, and they made sure that this doctor knew it. My mom yelled at the doctor in the middle of Children's Hospital, "You just watch, I am going to prove you wrong!" The doctor simply said, "I hope you do."

Since this was the 1970s, educational toy stores were extremely rare. But when you live about an hour and a half from Toronto, one of the biggest cities in the Western Hemisphere, there are plenty of specialty stores within a day's drive. My parents did everything to make sure that I was learning all the time. In addition to the use of educational toys, adults were not allowed to baby-talk me, and my parents spent countless hours mentally engaging me to make sure I was learning. Still within all that time spent working to learn, I was also showered in an endless fountain of love, encouragement, and support. I was lucky that my dad could provide so mom could stay at home to raise us. It is so amazing how hard she worked being a great mom, as she helped us to manage our current issues, and still work to prepare us for adulthood. The message in our house was clear and consistent: no matter what, always strive to be your best. We may not always win, but we always make sure we do everything possible to have success.

Many of my childhood and adolescent memories are cluttered with doctors, tests, and visits downtown to Children's Hospital. Even typing this now, I can remember the red carpet in the lobby where we walked in, that bizarre smell that wasn't quite hospital but was definitely very sanitary, and the cheery, almost saccharine-y wallpaper. I remember as a kid looking forward to seeing the woman who recorded my height and weight. When we would walk into the waiting room, this wonderful lady with the biggest smile you could ever imagine was always there. It felt as if she was waiting there just for me. I would run up to her and give her a huge hug that she returned with every ounce of love! I don't remember her name today, but I still remember that kind smile, and I know it was her kindness and affection that made the hospital so much less scary of a place. Instead of giving me shots and tests, she gave me hugs and lollipops; what more could a scared child ever ask for. Not to be outdone, I also remember Dr. M from the hospital. While she did have to give me shots and blood draws, her affection was very clearly communicated. She loved and cared about me so deeply that I would still visit her even after I was discharged from the hospital. I guess the lesson in that is that a little kindness goes a very long way with terrified patients of all ages!

Much like what I deal with today with Acromegaly, when I would go to the hospital for my semi-annual visits, my room was one of the most popular spots for the staff to visit. Doctors on duty, residents, nurses, and students would come in and ask me the same questions over and over. Even though meeting with all those medical people when I was a child was annoying, frustrating, and sometimes embarrassing, I hope that my efforts as a child helped to make today's children easier to treat.

As the years passed and I was more of a veteran of the Children's Hospital visits, I started to look forward to them because this was one of the few times during the year when people would be examining how different I was in order to be helpful to me, unlike my peers, who made me feel very uncomfortable about my size. Kids can be very cruel in school, and I was ill-equipped to deal with the vicious comments. As a young child I was always one of the shortest kids in my class; that is until summer break of sixth grade, when I came back as one of the tallest in my class. The abuse did not stop, it just changed. Now instead of the kids making fun of my being small, they started to pick on my being big. My first reaction was to use my new large size to intimidate kids, but that just did not fit my personality since no matter how physically large I grew, I always saw myself as average or small. More than that though, my parents raised us to believe that brains were more important than muscle, so I never got into more than a handful of confrontations before I decided to use humor to talk my way out of trouble. You can go very far in life if you can make people laugh, and this saved me from more fights than I would care to count.

As I grew into a teenager my thyroid was less of a problem, and I was discharged from the hospital after a few pubescent hospital examinations. Since the thyroid is a hormonal issue, knowing how I handled puberty was essential for the medical team to learn, but *extremely embarrassing to me*! Picture being a twelve-year-old kid and having strangers in lab coats walk into your hospital room to ask if you feel anything around girls, if you ever get erect, and if you ever touch yourself *there*. I can say from personal experience that it is humiliating beyond anything you could imagine! The one thing that did help prepare me was the fact that my mom knew what was coming and kind of warned me ahead of time. When it comes to medicine, honesty is essential. If a shot was going to hurt, my parents would tell me it would probably hurt but they would be there to hold my hand. If they didn't know, that is what they said. I really think that anticipating the pain hurts less than doubting your parents' reassurances. I know that I trusted my parents because they would always give me the best information they had. So when my parents would tell me the doctors were going to ask questions about physical development and I should just be as honest as possible, I trusted them. This helped me a great deal.

I guess having my thyroid issues as a teen prepared me for my issues as an adult: too many doctors, too many interviews, too many unknowns, and all the fear and exhaustion that comes from too many "too many's." I am not sure which diagnosis was tougher for our family: the Acromegaly or the thyroid, because while the thyroid was a new issue for the 1970s with no ability to do patient research, being told that you have a tumor in your head after you lost your dad to brain cancer will shake you to your core.

Medical Stress Hits the Family Again

It was November of 1994 when my dad was diagnosed with brain cancer. For the first time since I had been dealing with my thyroid, I was living and breathing medical appointments again. Wayne the family goofball suddenly had to act like the head of the family.

As children, our parents were fantastically warm and loving people, just as wonderful as any kid could ever ask for. They showed love and encouragement to me and my sister, and our home was always open to our friends as if they were part of the family. There were no secrets or taboos in our house; mom and dad encouraged us to ask questions (even the uncomfortable ones), to explore, and to take risks; and if something went awry, we could fix it—but we should always be willing to try. Sure, my parents made mistakes, but they always made sure that they erred on the side of love for their children and their desire to see us grow into strong adults. It was this strong bond of love and trust that helped us through some of the darkest points of my life.

I never got to know my father's father because he also died from brain cancer—a cancer that is not supposed to be generational; but he died at age fifty-five, and my dad was now diagnosed right after his fiftieth birthday. To say that fear shot through the entire family was an understatement. Immediately my family physician sent me for a battery of tests just to make sure there were no signs of anything. I had started to put on weight at the time, but it is tough to say whether it was the start of Acromegaly or the incredibly unhealthy diet that is involved with hospital life. Fried foods, heavy cheeses, chips, cookies, and soda pop in an almost endless supply made up my life, so the sudden weight gain was pretty easy to dismiss as my fault. The medical complaints I did have were non-specific enough as to be missed by several doctors.

Unfortunately, it would be easy for one or two specialist physicians to miss my diagnosis, with the wide-ranging issues I suffered with, many of which I didn't think to complain about.

Issues doctors did notice:

- massive weight gain: dismissed as lots of hospital cafeteria food and fast food
- colon polyps: tested for medical issues but dismissed as dietary issue
- anger, fatigue, snoring: attributed to stress from dealing with dad's medical issues and family management

Issues I did not know to discuss with doctors yet (but they are aware of now):

- tingling in extremities
- severe jaw pain: figured it was just a dental issue and I didn't want braces *again*
- facial change: blamed on weight gain

Issues I did not notice right away, or ignored:

- enlarged hands and feet
- headaches that I just kept taking aspirin for—I mean, why tell a doctor about a headache?!

One of the many difficulties of having a sick family member is that all personal and family problems are magnified. My dad was one of the most loving, affectionate people anyone could ever hope to know, so when he became sick it put stress on the whole family, and we were all ill-prepared to deal with it.

So when dad was diagnosed with brain cancer, sis was a teenager in college doing well. I however, was the grand old age of twenty-two, and struggling in Community College . . . my *second* attempt at higher level academics. I tried to take care of dad and go to school, but I found myself falling asleep in class and totally unable to focus.

I went to apologize to my professor and explain why I was falling asleep. She suggested that I withdraw from school to help take care of dad. I am very glad I heeded her advice. I took him to his appointments, sat with him, and took care of him as best I could. He did it for me when I was younger. This was the least I could do in return. From his first complaint of a backache in November, dad would have surgery on the Monday after the Super Bowl. I sat and ate pizza with him as I watched the game and he slept. I am still appreciative of mom's brilliance. This maudlin memory is still one of my lasting memories, since dad did teach me football. While dad was not sick for very long, passing on March 29, 1995, the stress of losing a family member put us all through hell. It was one of the definite turning points in my life—when things became less funny and I became more serious about everything. After my dad's illness and subsequent passing, the entire family suffered together… in a matter of speaking. See, my dad was a natural leader whose warmth could fill a room, and a kindness that made people eager to follow him. His nature was to be firm, but kind. Strong, but loving. Anyone who ever met him instantly fell in love with him. Even when he disagreed with people, he had a gentle quality about him that the correction was welcomed.

When my dad was diagnosed and traveling the cancer path, our family was tremendously on edge. It made for some very tense moments throughout the entire family, and since dad could not navigate the storm, what was bad became worse. There is no good side to the emotional stress that illness puts on a family. No matter how loving a family is, losing a loved one is hard. But if there are unresolved issues, regardless of whether you know they exist, no matter how far underground they appear to be, it is amazing how quickly tensions can bubble over.

When we got the diagnosis that my dad had cancer, it naturally tore us all apart emotionally! Mom wanted me and my sister to meet with the doctor so we could get our questions answered. The obvious first one was *"is my dad going to die?!"* The response was a less-than-confident "we don't think so." The time given was usually a decade or longer, depending on the doctor. Well, as we were driving home from the hospital on the night of diagnosis, preparing to basically move in to the hospital waiting room, mom asked me to call the important people, since she could not. It wasn't easy for me either, but I understood. Needless to say, reactions from everybody were off the charts! Words were inspired through fear, love, and confusion. Those are the words that can hurt most though… and they did. One thoughtless statement garnered a thoughtless response. And you could almost hear the announcer in the Vegas tuxedo, *Let's get ready to rumbllllllle!!!!!!!!* And sadly, everyone would arch their backs as the fight marched on and we all blindly marched towards the cliff. A family that was once as close as any family could ever hope to be was now fighting to tolerate each other's presence while in the same building. And it was all because we all just wanted the best for my dad. I wish I could say that I was not party to the bickering, but I was right there on the front lines—protecting family honor, I guess.

If my dad had lived the ten-plus years they had hoped, we probably would have kissed and made up before too much time had passed. Sadly, this was not to be the case. Four months of intense medications, surgery, and emotions does not provide a lot of recovery time for an injured family's wounds to heal. Rather, it would exacerbate emotional wounds, and make poor behavior worse.

Love can manifest itself in very different ways. It makes people act and say things they may not normally do or say, and it can drive the kindest people to say things they don't mean because they are sad, scared, or tense. The problem is that "sorry" is not a bandage, and there is no aspirin that can take away the power of negative words or poor behavior. Our family was definitely challenged by the illness and eventual passing of my father. With a conscious effort, our nuclear family unit grew intensely closer, but major ripples in the pond tore apart our more extended family. As the new "man of the family," I was trying to manage shifting from bachelor with no responsibilities to responsible adult, and that would be no easy task even with a perfectly normal life. On top of that, I was dealing with the stress of being parent to my middle-aged father, almost surrogate husband to my mother, and just to add to it all, my own emotions were out of control because of the beginnings of a yet undiagnosed disease.

The positive postscript to the family rift is that cooler heads would eventually prevail. My sister and my cousin worked for years to build the bridge, and their persistence would eventually lead to a détente in the family. In recent years, many of us have actually gotten past the point of friendly to even becoming family again. The overarching story here, and the reason I am sharing this, is simple. Many people who are reading this are probably struggling with your own family issues. Please, try to put your angry emotions aside. Don't let your anger at a disease steal even one moment with the people you love. You know you love the person that you are fighting with. In all likelihood, your anger is directly connected to your love for the person and the fear of a cruel disease. Don't let your love be a casualty of war as it relates to some stupid disease! Trust me, words hurt for a very long time, and you need each other now more than ever!

This Sounds Weird, but My Jaw Hurts!

Somewhere soon after dad's diagnosis and eventual passing, I started to notice symptoms related to my Acromegaly, but didn't actually know they meant anything. I remember the first problem that was significant enough to say out loud. It was only a few months after dad passed and our little nuclear family (mom, sis, and myself) had worked to reshape our lives together. One of our efforts included making an effort to go out for lunch on Saturday afternoons. Mom and I were in the car one sunny spring day as we were driving to lunch. The radio was on in the background filling the spaces of our awkward conversations of nothingness. The unwritten mission was to fill the silence so we didn't actually have to talk about the twenty-four-hour anguish we had just survived. In between vacant conversations about the weather, politics, or whatever else we could think of, I asked my mom if it was possible for my lower jaw to hurt again, more than a decade after finishing a full course of orthodontia. I don't really know why I asked her, she was not a dentist; I guess the Dr. Mom idea was just another great way to keep us distracted. At the end of the day, when you don't like going to real dentists, it is easier to talk to Dr. Mom, especially when she is equally or more terrified of dentists. Her reply was that it was probably nothing, but if I was worried I should go to the dentist to get things checked out. I immediately flashed back to my adolescence in the orthodontist's chair. *Sitting and wondering about the weird smell in the room as I looked at a clay impression of my teeth, hoping that maybe he forgot I was there. But, alas, he had not. Like a bad dream, suddenly the doctor appeared in the room, white hair, white coat, and a hunched back. I always wondered if he got that from torturing kids all day long. It is not like I pitied him for his back. Hell, maybe if he didn't spend his career constantly trying to shove both hands and both feet into my mouth at the same time, he would be able to stand better!* Ha! Dentist? No way! I made some jokes that I would go to the dentist right after mom did; we shared some giggles and the conversation vanished into some other empty discussion.

The years would pass on like this. Saturdays became mom, me, and sis for lunch. Not always all three of us, but some combination of the three. This would become more complicated as I decided to go back to college in August 2000, a decision I didn't really enter into lightly. Even though I was twenty-seven years old and horribly uncomfortable with just about every aspect of my being, I plodded forward, in spite of the doubters. In fact, when I told one of my closest confidantes I was considering the return to college, he told me to keep it quiet: "That way, when you fuck it up again, no one can throw it up in your face!" Hmm . . . this was quite the reputation I had built for myself. The first time I walked into a classroom in college, someone asked me about the class. She thought I was the professor. *Ugh, this could be ugly.*

The impetus for this decision to return to college was easy. I had a car accident about 30 months previous, when I was working in sales. I did well enough in business-to-business sales, but never really enjoyed it. I guess it was because I never felt like I was doing anything that benefitted anyone but my boss. This is not to condemn the profession of sales as a whole; but it was frustrating to me in large part because, as a result of the car accident, I bulged two discs in my lower back, causing unimaginable pain on a twenty-four-hour basis. Since the career was worsening the back, the career got the blame. After the accident I took several months to recover before I forced myself back to work. But since I never fully healed from the accident, I ended up in a situation where I had trouble holding a job for too many months in a row. This was not because I didn't work hard enough, but because I worked so hard that eventually my back would knock me out for several days. Two days on, three days off is not the life of a successful salesman. I was starting to have visions of my life as Willy Loman from *Death of a Salesman*, the man who basically worked himself to death. Of course, at least he had a career with one company; so I guess Willy had a life that was still enviable to me. But this was a fate that I wanted no part of, and the reevaluation of my situation led me back to school.

As if the stress of returning to college as a twenty-seven-year-old freshman wasn't enough for the average person to handle, the yet-undiagnosed Acromegaly was in full swing. I was starting to gain weight, my back was still in pain, and I was chronically exhausted. Every time I went to the doctor I complained about how lousy I felt, but it was either dismissed with a pill or a shrug of indifference. The doctors would send me for tests that would come back negative, send me for other tests that were also fine, and then finally look at me with eyes that said I was a hypochondriac. It was then that they generally informed me that they couldn't help because my challenges were related to lifestyle. I was working lousy jobs to pay the bills for a full time education which caused a total lack of sleep from overwork, which led to poor dietary habits, which explained the weight gain, which explained the physical pain, which led to poor sleeping patterns, which led to feeling lousy all the time. I was trapped in a horrible cycle of negativity that was my own doing, according to the doctors.

Doc, I Just Feel Lousy

It is difficult to describe how I was feeling so it makes sense to someone who has never dealt with the symptoms of Acromegaly, but I always just *felt bad*. It felt like my limited free time between school and work was spent seeing my doctor, just trying to get his attention. I was almost constantly complaining of back and joint pain, chronic exhaustion, and always feeling angry. He would respond by occasionally sending me for blood work, but all tests came back negative. The only test that kept coming back badly was my thyroid. It seemed like every time I got my blood drawn, my synthetic thyroid prescription would go up again. I was almost afraid that if I donated blood, the doctor would call me with a new prescription dosage! At its highest dosage, my synthetic thyroid prescription reached over *five times* the average dosage for an adult male of my age, but I was still complaining about being tired all the time, and the doctor kept saying that nothing was physically wrong with me. Clearly my doctor and I were at an impasse. But since he had the diplomas and the authority blessed to him by wearing a lab coat with his name monogrammed on the pocket, I was always going to be wrong. In hindsight, I guess the doctor was right, in a way. After all, the problem *really was all in my head.*

The Storm That Strikes without Any Warning

The biggest problem I struggled with before my Acromegaly diagnosis was the unpredictable emotions. The best way I can describe my emotional instability was that it was like a tornado going through a trailer park; while the incident may only last for moments, the after-effects take far longer to repair. And by the time the 2000s had rolled in, I was positively volatile. I could barely stand myself, so I don't know how the rest of the world did!

A typical Saturday family lunch is difficult to represent because they became less typical as the anger would make me somewhat unpredictable. The thing about the Acro-anger for me is that it is an all-encompassing, full-body anger that would literally take over my entire persona. There doesn't need to be a rational reason for the anger. Hell, most of the times that my anger got the best of me, even I wasn't entirely sure why I was so angry! Ironically, this only made it worse. I would watch Wayne losing control almost like a bad television show, and I didn't like angry-Wayne; but I had no idea what was bringing him on, or why; so I would get angrier trying to stem the tide of anger without any tools with which to do it. It wasn't just family that got to see this. I was no better with my friends. We could be sitting, laughing, and having a good time and for no reason my brain would get angry and I would go into this tornado of raw fury because I had no idea what was going on or how to control it. I mean, why would my brain make me angry unless it had a good reason?

So while I was battling my own emotional stability, without understanding why I was so angry, life went on as usual. I started student teaching in 2002, but my body didn't care that I had other, more pressing issues to deal with than being emotionally crippled by a pit of a tumor I didn't know existed! My emotions were no more stable at work than they were anywhere else. Even as a student teacher, practicing the new skills I was so excited to try out, these emotions would occasionally get the best of me. When I was a young student, I always responded best to the teachers who were the most entertaining, so that was what I wanted to be; the fun teacher. As a teacher, I always tried to use humor to help children understand material better. Learning is easier while laughing than while yawning. Unfortunately, no one in the classroom, including myself, could really predict my emotional issues because, simply put, before diagnosis, my brain frequently betrayed all of us. I would be in the middle of teaching new material and would make a joke that the students would laugh at, but with my hyper-sensitive brain, if they started to laugh for a time that I thought was too long, I would react like they were laughing at me, and not with me; and I would become utterly unglued and yell at a very confused classroom of children. After I yelled, the students would immediately quiet down, but there would be a sea of mystified faces. And frankly, I was as confused, frustrated, and saddened as they were. This was probably the most trying part of my life before diagnosis. I knew I had no control over my emotions, but had no clue why I was feeling like that, or how to reestablish control, which frustrated and angered me, which further fed the beast. To hate the person in the mirror is a very isolating emotion.

Finally Someone Tells Me I Have a Real Problem

A strange relief finally came in November of 2004, a relief that brought a whole new world of unknowns. My general practitioner officially threw his hands up in exasperation after a new series of blood work showed that even though I still complained about being tired and irritable, everything was fine, except that my thyroid was still low. I was already up to 525 mcg, which was far beyond normal for an adult male, and it was going up?! Something was clearly not right, and it was finally time for me to see an endocrinologist who could better explore my complaints.

It was a cold, snowy day as I sat in the endo's parking lot. As I was snuffing out a cigarette, I was just thinking how irritating it was that I had to see another doctor. It just seemed like another opportunity for another expert to call me crazy... *and why can't I kick this disgusting habit?! Whatever. I'll quit tomorrow. Let's get this over with.*

After the nurse weighed me, I told her that I normally don't weight 326; it's my wallet, my boots, the scale, the air in the room was heavy, or anything else I could blame. The nurse gave a slightly condescending smile and escorted me back to the far part of this medical office. Long gone were the days of Children's Hospital, but for the first time since I was a teenager I was going to see an endocrinologist. This just feels weird. "Hi, Wayne, my name is Howard," he said as he almost eagerly burst in the room. It was such a difference from the black cloud I felt hanging over my head that one couldn't help but notice the contrasting atmosphere in the room. After shaking my hand, he made a comment about its size, but this was nothing new to me. I am used to the hand jokes, and I think I have heard them all by now. Baseball glove, banana hands, sausage fingers . . . just to name a few. Anyway, he asked me why I was there in a way that actually sounded like he genuinely cared. After I started listing symptoms, you could tell his brain started whirring. I was lethargic and irritable, and I felt like I was falling apart. Before he even knew how much thyroxine I was on, I warned him not to lower it. *They have tried lowering the dosage before, and I get worse... so you had better not change anything!* I was waiting for the rolling eyes or some hint of annoyance that I had seen by so many medical people before, but happily Dr. L was simultaneously reassuring and scientific—not an easy pair to pull off. You could tell he had a grip on my issue, and his radiating confidence and sympathy was a welcome change in my weary existence. He evenly stated that he would not change anything until we had a better idea of what was going on, and I breathed a huge sigh of relief; *finally someone gets it!*.

Then, almost without warning, he let go with a stream of questions like I hadn't seen since my days at Children's Hospital! *Have I noticed any changes in my body size, am I having trouble sleeping, have I noticed a change in my sexuality, have I noticed any tingling in my arms or legs?* Pretty strange questions, but I answered as honestly as I could, even though I was silently dying from embarrassment, especially about my sexuality. *At 6'3", 326 pounds, working lousy jobs to pay the bills, and a miserable attitude, how could I possibly know if my sexuality was off?* I guess saying there was no change was the truth—I wanted women who didn't want me. No change. The questions mercifully ended, and Dr. L informed me that he thought he knew exactly what was wrong, and that it was treatable. Without exaggeration, tears filled my eyes. "You mean I am not crazy? What's wrong with me?" In hindsight, I am glad he said we needed to wait until the results were definite but there was no reason to worry before we knew for sure. I left the doctor's office with orders for what he called "the gold standard" in diagnosis. *Real medical tests beyond testing my thyroid? This was different . . . and anything different was good!* Finally I felt like a ray of hope was shining down on me and that someday I might feel better.

I ran out to the car and called to immediately schedule the blood test and the MRI for as quickly as possible. The sooner I could get in for the tests, the sooner Dr. L could put me on the road to health. It would take a week to get it all done, but everything finally got finished.

The tests were rough, but I got through them. I hate MRIs. Trapped in a metal tube for an hour for essentially two tests: one normal and one with contrast. With contrast is a really polite way to say NUCLEAR DYE!!! I was having visions of Chernobyl and Three Mile Island flowing through my veins, and was pretty amused by it. Hell, at least I was laughing a little—a new emotion indeed. As it turned out, the dye actually felt kind of cool going in, until you realize that there is *nuclear dye streaming through your body.* The blood test was the next stop, and it was no fun either. Blood draws at 0 minutes, then at 20, 40, 60, 90, and 120 minutes are not much fun, but what's even worse are the looks from others in the waiting room when you walk right past them to get your blood drawn.

Oh, who am I kidding… I thought the sneering faces were kind of funny. Regardless, for the first time in my life I knew what the beer keg feels like!

Waiting for the test results seemed to take forever, but finally the day of mixed blessing was upon me. It was the most bizarre feeling of Christmas morning mixed with mortal dread! Excitement, anticipation, and abject fear were jockeying for position as my primary emotion.

Another bitter cold Buffalo afternoon, going into evening. It felt like my life was stuck in the plot of some cheesy B-movie and the director loved weather symbolism, using cold and gray as the redundant theme.

I got out of the car and stomped out what would come to be my last ever cigarette. I walked into the office and scanned the lobby. Why is everyone there? Diabetes? Check up? Wondering how many have been waiting ten years for their diagnosis.

The nurse called my name and it almost felt like I could feel an echo in the hollowness of her voice. We walked back to the room as I tried to look cool. I waited patiently in the room, or at least attempting the veneer of patience, thumbing through a magazine without really noticing any of the words on the page or really even being able to keep a thought in my head. Finally Dr. L walked in, as pleasant as ever, and said that he was right; we knew what was wrong. "You have a tumor in your head, but it is not cancer." I wish I could say I heard anything but the words *tumor* and *cancer*, but my heart sunk to my feet and my eyes filled instantly with tears. All I could hear was Charlie Brown's teacher talking to me after that. I know he was talking, telling me that the tumor was in my pituitary, and it was not cancerous but did require immediate treatment. We went over the next steps—meeting with a neurosurgeon and starting immediately on medication, after the insurance approved it. If I said I was half-listening, I would be overstating it. Immediately my brain went into overdrive, rapidly firing questions to my subconscious that I couldn't possibly answer: How do I tell my family? What do I tell my family? What the hell is going on with me? How much time do I have? *Am I going to die?* Finally Dr. L stopped talking and asked me if I had any questions. My brain screamed YES! But the line of questions in my head was so bottlenecked that nothing came out, and I just kind of shrugged a dejected no. I know he said something encouraging before he left, but I have no idea what it was. *I have a tumor. Something is growing inside my head. What do I say to my family?*

As if someone writing the book of my life just decided to start a new chapter, the doctor walked out to get some forms and information so I could start my new life path as a person with a tumor. Dizzied by hyperperception of my surroundings, I was overly aware of all the inconsequential nuances of a doctor's office like the brightness of the lights, the magazines askew on the chair, and a bunch of the doctor's doodles on the exam table paper cover. The nurse walked in, took off the butcher paper, and in a sweet voice told me how great the doctor was because he would sit with me until I understood everything. She was right, Dr. L was pretty great, but my mind was elsewhere. I wished I could scream, or cry, whatever… But now I had to face the rest of my universe. It was about ten years before that we had lost dad to brain cancer, and now I had to try to explain all this? Saying I was totally overwhelmed would be an understatement.

I got to the car, still in a daze. I stared at my phone and tried to decide what to do… Looking at my cell phone like the first caveman to discover fire, I finally assembled my wits enough to dial the phone. "Hi, Nikki, are you still at work?" I would nervously ask my sister. "Yeah, but I'm getting ready to leave." I asked her to wait, that there was something I NEEDED to talk with her about. Since we weren't all that social with each other at the time, I guess my tone and urgency told her that I had something significant to tell her.

As I drove, I kept having the conversation in my brain, trying to figure out what I was going to say. I knew she was going to have the same questions I did. I walked in to her place of work and summoned every ounce of energy I had to make my way through the building with a straight face. When I got to her office, I closed the door behind me and told her the whole story. I was listening to myself tell the story and almost lost it when I heard tumor again. It's like every time I heard the word it became more real. Both of us unsure, afraid, and sad, we immediately started reliving the loss of dad and all the what if's. The obvious next question was how do I tell mom?! We both thought straightforward was best. But I was dreading telling her. Mom was not all too healthy, and she didn't need this stress!

Much to my surprise at the time, mom would be the pillar of strength and the voice of reason we all needed to push through. When we were children my mom was one of the most energetic, happy people I have ever met. All that changed after she fell and injured her back in the mid-1980s. After numerous back surgeries, she was slowed down, considerably. And then, in 1990, the doctors were convinced she had lymphoma, but it turned out to *only* be Sarcoidosis, a rare lung disease that was slowly eating her away from the inside, out. Still struggling with the Sarcoid, she had lost dad, her life-mate, to brain cancer only five years later. How much more could this woman be asked to handle?

Much to my very pleasant surprise, she would be the one to readjust my brain. Big brave Wayne could not even get through the whole story without getting weepy. Thankfully, no matter how infirmed mom was, when she was needed, she could always rise to an occasion. Once I was done talking, she asked me a few frank questions that I did not know the answers to: was I going to die, is this curable, how is this going to affect my life? I kept saying I don't know, and her reaction was simple and blunt, but said with the love that only a mother could offer at such a time. "Before we get nervous about what might happen, let's find out more about what is going to happen." This made sense, and it helped to calm me a lot. I knew this already, but I was too emotionally invested to see this obvious response. There is nothing like a mom when the chips are down.

Talking to the Rest of the Crew

Phew! I got through telling mom and sis. Now to tell other family and friends. I guess I could have kept it quiet, but I just had to let it out. I was so enveloped with my own fears that staying quiet would have been a near impossibility.

In a weird way, there was a catharsis in sharing. Like every time I heard myself telling people about it, I would get more used to the diagnosis. I mean, I was still scared as hell about the endless unknowns, and I still wasn't entirely convinced I wouldn't die, but I was getting better at knowing the information.

One of the things I remember about this point in my life was feeling an obligation to indulge people's good intentions as I was showered in oceans of free medical advice from well-meaning people. While I appreciated the affection that manifested itself as unsolicited advice, it wasn't what I needed at the time. I am not sure I knew what I needed, but now I understand. We want a strong shoulder and a good ear. If you have a loved one struggling with a big diagnosis, please don't feel a need to fill awkward silence with sage advice. We have already been diagnosed, and that awkward silence you hear is us thinking. We already have enough medical professionals shoving enough data in our brains. Don't be another expert, just be a good friend. If someone has been diagnosed with a major illness, the best thing you can say is "oh man, I am so truly sorry! Let's go do ____ this weekend." And just fill in the blank with whatever is normal. Trust me, all we want is a sense of normalcy. Just ask how things are. If we want to talk, we will. But if we want to talk about something else, that is equally healthy. Sometimes we need a break from our medical issues. When you just sit and listen and make us laugh, it is more appreciated. This is why they are called *necessary* distractions!

The advice given out of love can be quite taxing to the patient's ear. When I was first diagnosed, I was already so overwhelmed with people sharing their "brilliance" that I could scream! Ever try to take a drink from a firehose? Get it? After I was diagnosed I was told to try herbs, to look online to make sure the doctor is right, *to be positive to be able to defeat this disease*, and on and on and on. I did not want to get mad at the people who cared enough to try to help, but I also did not want to be told that I needed to be positive, especially when this instruction came within twenty-four hours of being diagnosed. I knew I had to be positive, but I was just diagnosed and I was pissed off. More than that, I wanted to be pissed off for a little while… in fact, I felt damn *entitled* to be pissed off! I would be positive in a week . . . maybe two. Just give me time to rage first. Please!

As a newly diagnosed patient, no matter how many friends or family members that loved and cared for me, I still felt like I was totally alone in my battle. The couch in my family room was sitting under a water stain on the ceiling. Today I could still draw that exact stain from memory because of the endless hours I spent staring at it. Not really thinking or doing anything. The television could be on, the stereo could be cranked up, people could be over. I still felt totally alone; all the time. I was pretty sure I could feel the tumor inside my head. When I would actually stop to think about it, the sentence almost become a mantra: "oh my god, there is something growing inside me." Hell, I hated looking in a mirror because I was convinced I could see the thing growing. No one has advice to help counteract that emotion. Just love us in spite of our imperfections.

Reality Sinks In

As Thanksgiving 2004 turned towards New Year's 2005, reality started to sink in and I knew I had to deal with it. The first thing I thought I needed to do was something I had never done before with a medical issue: go online in search of information. I never wanted to be someone who would be a double-click backseat driver for everything the doctor said, but what I did want was to cure the feelings of isolation and frustration.

I've learned over the course of my life travels that fear and loneliness manifest in one of two primary directions, and sometimes in simultaneous fashion. These two directions are woeful sadness and bitter anger! So I figured that if I could learn something about what I was dealing with, maybe I would be able to control the frustrations of the unknown. I went to look up Acromegaly online, but with my swiss cheese brain, that was more of an adventure than it should have been. I had no idea what the name of my disease was, which made research *slightly* more difficult. I am glad that search engines have the ability to say, "Hey, dummy, I think you mean…," but whatever I typed in was such a mess that I could almost see the search engine shrug and say "If you're going to make up words, I am not going to help you!" In hindsight, the message may have been a little different than that, but that was what I felt like it said. Annoyed with myself for forgetting how to spell the name of the disease, I called the doctor's office and stupidly asked the receptionist, "What is the name of my disease again?!" Armed with the right word and correct spelling, I sauntered off on my quest of knowledge… only to be turned back again! I searched and searched but largely came up dry. There was one message board that was almost completely dormant, and when there were posts, they were so depressing. Other websites about the disease were either owned by medical companies or looked like they were. The information was very complicated and did nothing to answer my more basic questions as a patient. Even with these limited tools, or maybe because of them, I felt even more frustrated than before. I guess I have to try to listen better the next time I go to the doctor.

My follow-up appointment with the endocrinologist came more quickly than I could imagine. For the follow-up visit, mom insisted on going with me. As someone who is staunchly independent, I was having none of that, but mom was absolutely correct. Because I was so emotionally invested, mom was able to hear information that I was too overwhelmed to catch. Dr. L said recovery from surgery could be several weeks, but I knew I couldn't get that kind of time off since I had just started a new job teaching. I would have to wait until summer break. So he told me that we would start with the simplest medication, just to get treatment started. "And hopefully it will even shrink the tumor to make the surgery easier!" I was going to be starting on an injectable medication that I would need to put into my belly three times a day. I guess the panic was written all over my face because mom, who was diabetic, assured me she could help me learn how to self-inject. In addition to the injections, I got a referral to see a neurosurgeon. "Really? I am so young and now I have a *neurosurgeon?! This cannot be real. I am just stuck in a bad dream!"* I wasn't though. I was really going to see a neurosurgeon, and he was really in charge of navigating the next major steps of my healthcare path.

The Path from Diagnosis to Surgery . . . A Very Long Road

I have been very lucky in my life that most of the people I have surrounded myself with have been good people, but even the kindest, most well-intended person can say things that will drive a person's emotions 30 miles around the bend.

When I called the neurosurgeon's office for the first time, I was on pins and needles. I asked for an appointment to see Dr. X and the nurse asked me if I was a returning patient. When I said no, she informed me that new patient appointments were booking 3 months out. Well, if that is what it is, then that is what will have to be. She then asked what my diagnosis was; why did I need a neurosurgeon? My response was one word: Acromegaly. "Oh. How is this Tuesday at 10:00 a.m.?" It was Friday. *I just got put to the front of the list by this disease?! Wow, that's so cool!* Then, it hit me two seconds later… *what is the endocrinologist not telling me? Am I going to die if I don't have this surgery immediately? What is happening to me?* While this nurse was simply trying to help me, the urgency in her voice and my ignorance added up to one big anxiety attack! Fear of the unknown is very easy for new patients, and I had more than my fair share of nerves. It is amazing how easily your mind wanders to a worst-case scenario when thrust into such a high-stakes vortex.

The nurse sent me the forms that needed to be filled out in advance and as soon as I opened the envelope it was like a punch to the jaw. There it was on the letterhead: my father's neurosurgeon was part of this firm. Another reminder of brain cancer while navigating my own tumor troubles. The paperwork then asked me about my family medical history, and within the list of over 20 different medical conditions, I checked more than half. *Wow, I really lost at genetic roulette!*

Before I knew it, Tuesday was upon us, and I was at the surgeon's office; alone again. I looked around the room wondering how many other people were going there for brain surgery. Another doctor's office with more outdated magazines where I could pretend to read about bass fishing or how to best furnish my cottage, or articles about sporting events that happened half a decade ago. *The things I do to blend in.* I was finally invited back for the meeting I was nervously anticipating. As the nurse checked me in, she asked if I would meet their student physician assistant. This is not new; in fact, ever since diagnosis, meeting the student seems like part of the doctor visit. This is totally up to the patient, but I figured that this helps future patients, so I kind of have a duty. The student came in and asked the typical questions about symptoms, physical impacts, emotions, and the rest of the drill. You could almost see her mentally cross-referencing her textbooks… until the surgeon *blasted* into the room. He introduced himself, said I definitely had Acromegaly and needed transsphenoidal surgery, handed me a pamphlet, told me to schedule an appointment for surgery, said that if the surgery failed we could always do Gamma Knife, asked if I had any questions, and ran out. Even if I had any questions, I don't think he was actually in there long enough to hear them. In fact, I am not sure that he took a breath during our entire visit.

And now the clock had started. Countdown for surgery was upon us. The surgeon agreed with Dr. L, my endo, that the surgery could wait until school had ended. The interval might actually be beneficial for shrinking the little bugger because, as I would come to learn, my tumor had grown in an "L" shape around my carotid artery. This simply meant that the likelihood of actually removing the whole thing surgically was no more than 25%. Better odds than any casino, but I don't like to gamble my paycheck, much less my life!

I asked Dr. L if it was worth doing the surgery, and he said it was totally up to me. *Well of course, I already know that! But am I wasting my time if they can't get the whole thing out?* I took his somewhat frustrating non-response and repackaged it. "Dr. L, if I were a member of your family and I was asking for advice, what would you tell me to do?" Well, something clicked with that. For the first time in our relationship, he stopped dead in his tracks. Finally I gave him a question that he really needed to ponder! He thought and thought, and then said that no one had ever asked him a question in such a way. He thought about it for probably about 20 seconds, which felt hours to me. He finally said that he would probably recommend the surgery because the risk of surgical complications was very small, and if it did fail we would at least have removed a lot of the tumor in the process. "Sounds good to me doc." After the appointment ended, we were walking and chatting to the front and I passively added, "Like Dr. X said, if the surgery fails, there is always Gamma Knife too." Dr. L's reaction was positively visceral. He grabbed my arm and dragged me into an empty office. This was totally out of character for him, so he definitely had my attention now. When Dr. X had mentioned Gamma Knife, my mind immediately had flashes of *Star Wars* running through it. *I was mentally transported to being 7 years old in the big theater with my dad and me eating popcorn. Memories that good could only be good, right?* So instead of doing any research, I told myself "wow! That sounds so cool!" Dr. L snapped me back to the reality of medicine, saying that if I ever did Gamma Knife he would refuse to treat me ever again. *What? Why?!* Because, he explained, the potential damage to other parts of my pituitary was too extreme. Since I already had thyroid issues, the risk of needing several more medications was too high. Unlike the surgery, my risk with Gamma Knife was just not worth the reward. When I got home that night, intellectual curiosity got the best of me, and I searched online for videos about Gamma Knife surgery. Those pleasant images of *Star Wars* and my dad were quickly eviscerated. Left in their place were visions of having a metal halo drilled into my skull and two hours of radiation. Dr. L was right; I was not a good candidate for Gamma Knife, emotionally if not medically. That night was one of the nights where it would have been nice to have had someone special in my life. Unfortunately, dating relationships were not my forte during this time. Relationships are difficult enough to manage with two healthy people.

On the night before surgery, I was obsessing over my own mortality. Sure, I'd had surgery before; but I was fifteen, and that was a sinus scraping. Yes, the surgery was in the same general area, but the two surgeries are similar the way that elementary t-ball and the World Series are both baseball. I spent the night before surgery walking through the neighborhood. Nowhere in particular. I was just walking around the neighborhood looking at the moon, seeing the lights in homes that were on at and three and four o' clock in the morning; wondering why they would be awake at this stupid hour. I knew what was causing my insomnia! *I may as well be awake now, in case I don't survive the surgery.*

The hospital on the morning of surgery was good enough. My family was walking on eggshells around me. I sensed it, and I guess in hindsight, I appreciate it. I feel badly how difficult I was to live with and be around, but now that I understand the correlation between Acro and temper, I do try to make sure I manage it well. The hospital staff was fantastic! Everyone was incredibly kind, and the anesthesiologist was amazing! I guess he saw how nervous I was about the surgery. After they gave me the sedative, I was the happiest guy in the building . . . but I still was visibly rattled when he brought the gas mask over. So he put it next to my mouth. He told me it was not on, and he would let me know before he turned it on. This eased my fears... and then I was surrounded by my family in ICU. I know they say that you have to wake up in recovery, but I swear I do not remember it!

My stay at the hospital was unadventurous, except for the fact that I knew I wanted to go home, and I knew immediately that I felt better. When I woke up the morning after surgery, I felt so much better that when Dr. L came to check on me, I started to cry tears of happiness!

The only complaint I had with the hospital stay was the fact that I really realized just how alone I was. Sure, friends and family stopped by. But not having a spouse, or even a girlfriend... I don't think it is lonelier than in the hospital after a major surgery. Of course, it is not like I was the best candidate for a relationship before surgery. I was quick to temper, could mow through a buffet restaurant, and was filled with self-loathing. Not exactly the ideal catch for a young woman … or old woman … or really any woman!

Trying to Manage Dating

On the relationship front, there have been several women who passed through my life over the years. No one was really close enough to me to ever be there to help through the innumerable doctor visits or major life-changing decisions. Plenty who said that they would have been there, *had they only known*. The problem I found with that statement was that it was their cue to depart at full sprint. I think that everyone wants to think they will always be the best versions of themselves, but it is a great deal of work to be that person.

I feel somewhat awkward discussing failed relationships here because I always seemed to be attracted to the worst person for me and my Acromegaly issues. As a human balance sheet, I had a lot of plusses but several glaring minuses too. Yes, I had my own home and eventually a good and stable job. With my master's degree, I had a bright future. But on the negative side, I was morbidly obese, I was always achy, and I had two distinct self-images. One was almost so negatively distorted that I didn't even know how to accept a compliment with a simple "thank you," and the other was so tremendously hyper-inflated that I really thought I was something incredible. In hindsight, both self-images were horribly wrong! But since you tend to attract exactly what you put out to the world, the people who I dated or tried to date had the same esteem issues I had.

Before I returned to college, I was not dating much. Not that I didn't want to, but I was a workaholic with confidence issues and a huge stomach. At my peak, I was 6'3" and maxed out at 330+ pounds, almost none of which was muscle. I was the guy who would go to buffets every night for dinner if I could have. I remember one time I was going to go for a Chinese buffet lunch, but I only had an hour for lunch, so I decided to go another time when I could actually enjoy a complete meal there. Needless to say, my physique was not exactly going to get me noticed for positive reasons. And if that was not enough, my emotions were already somewhat unstable from the yet-to-be-diagnosed tumor. In this section, I want to focus on two women that I really allowed to get very close to me: one from right before college and the other from right before (and after) diagnosis. As they say on television, any names mentioned have been changed to protect the innocent (and the guilty). It is sort of strange to discuss dating here because, while there were plenty of issues of negativity, a failed relationship includes responsibility by all parties involved.

The last woman I dated right before returning to college was Karen. I met her at work in 1999. She had a sense of humor that could cut a person to shreds before they even knew what happened to them. Since I tended towards sarcasm, I thought she was really funny, and she thought the same of me. On top of that, I thought that she was very good looking and she seemed to be equally attracted to me. That was enough to keep me interested. Our time together was short before she talked with me about moving in. It was a Baltimore Colts–style move after her roommate went to work. We got everything into one truck move with my neighbor's help. He asked me if I knew what I was doing because she didn't seem all that trustworthy; but of course I knew better. I was going to save her. We lasted a few months before things went totally sour. She kept needing just a few bucks here and there before it added into the thousands of dollars. I had to move out of town for work. She was going to join me, but when we went to the city to scout it out, she spent the entire time complaining, pointing out how stupid I was, and slamming doors any time we were at "home" and I wanted to hang out. Needless to say, when I pulled out of town, she did not follow. Probably the best thing for everyone.

When I returned to college, my life focus changed in just about every way. Yes, my career took a major U-turn. But I also discovered that the A-type personality was only one part of who I was. Yes, when it comes to my career, I need everything to be perfect. If you talk with just about anyone who has ever worked with me, I was always the hardest worker. My belief was that if I was the best at what I was doing, everyone else would want to be the best they could, and in turn, everything would be far more likely to be successful! Well, I learned in college that I needed to find someone that would let me get off the stage from time to time.

I met Michelle in 2001, halfway through my bachelor's program, and I knew she was different. We had an interesting relationship, where our lives would cross paths several times over the next nine years. Our relationship started off with a boom in 2001. The chemistry was obvious. We just fit together with ease; but it ended almost as quickly as it ignited when her abusive ex-boyfriend literally took her away from me, and she was afraid to fight back. I was sad to lose her, but I had no idea how to help step in and not make the abuse worse. Plus, we had just met. How was I realistically going to step in to such a situation? I backed off, hesitantly. In hindsight, I guess I subscribed to the "if you love something, set it free" mentality. Oddly enough, our paths would haphazardly cross again.

About nine months after the sudden departure, I was studying in Europe when I saw a statue that made me think of Michelle, so I emailed her. Disappointed but not surprised, she never responded. Then she would write back to a dormant e-mail account several months later, and I never got that message. Finally, and I really don't remember how, we managed to connect again in about 2005. The conversation picked up like we had never missed a day, and I was happy to hear that she was past the abusive ex, but was sad to hear that she was moving out of the country. *Oh well, our timing was never meant to be. But we can still be social, right?* Our first conversations were kind of dark, as we finally got to talk openly and honestly about our horror stories. She told me her stories of abuse that I couldn't even comprehend, and I told her all about my surgeries, tests, exams, and all the rest. I told her how I wanted to be there to help her, and she kept telling me that had she known about the surgeries, she would have been there for me, and I really wanted to believe her. Realistically, I knew that we both cared about each other but really had no way of really helping each other. I had no clue how to help her, and if she couldn't leave that guy to stop her own awful reality, my surgery certainly didn't stand a chance of getting in between them. Our friendship lasted for several weeks before the instant messaging/email relationship would die once again. There developed a pattern of our relationship that became pretty obvious to me. I tried to show her that I was a good guy and wanted to treat her extremely well, but I would go overboard. Couple that with her own understandable insecurities, and she did not know how to deal with it. In my reality, I saw her perspective of our relationship in a vicious cycle:

1. I love you.
2. I need you.
3. You are too needy, get away.

The final meet up and break up between me and Michelle would happen in 2008 when she was living about an hour away from me. We started talking again, and as usual, things were quite natural, but I tried to care too much, and she wasn't ready. After about two or three months of the cycle, we were both very frustrated with each other. She was in stage 3 of the "need" cycle at the time, and I hadn't heard from her in two weeks. I sent her an email saying I missed her and wanted to spend some time with her. Well, the reaction was one of pure fury. I was told that I was too clingy, I was suffocating her, I was manipulating her… and on, and on, and on. She told me she needed time, and I said that was fine; I was going to spend the evening with friends and we would talk in the morning. Over the course of the evening she sent me forty-seven texts, each one more demeaning and offensive than the previous one. The last of the messages complained that I would use my disease as an excuse every time I was having a bad day. If ever a person knew how to cause pain, it was Michelle. I am not sure if her hostility was malicious, a personality flaw, or a defense mechanism against previous life experiences. I am not really sure which one of those is most preferable. In hindsight, we both had our issues, but since our paths did keep crossing, I do have to take my share of the blame too. The emotional craziness that is Acromegaly can drive a person with the disease crazy, so it takes a very sensitive, loving couple to work past all of the hard spots. I think that, in spite of our harried past, Michelle will always have a soft spot in my heart. Whether or not we ever talk again, I guess time will tell.

Over the course of my managing Acro, I have become an expert at first and second dates, but not much past that. As a single man, I have no answers as to when to mention the disease to a new girlfriend. If I mention it too early, the woman heads for the door because I am broken, and who needs a guy who is unhealthy?! But if I mention it too late, I am withholding and cut off. Managing relationships and illness is a difficult line. I would love to say that I have figured out the mystery, but that would be a lie. My favorite first date story was a girl who was introduced to me as a friend of a friend. Nice woman, fun personality, and we seemed to have a lot in common. During one of our early chats, I had recently found out I was getting an award from my undergraduate college. Graduate of the Last Decade! I was so proud I stupidly told her. The reason that was stupid, you ask? Well, then I had to explain why I was getting the award, which led to my talking about my work with Acromegalics across the globe. I love everyone in this group and am in awe of how much support members of Acromegaly Community provide each other, but she stopped hearing when I told her I had the tumor. I knew when she stopped listening too. Trust me, you can hear it if you are paying enough attention. Two days later she called me to apologize and say we should go on a date. I, of course, said sure! Well, this date felt more like a doctor's appointment. No matter what I talked about, she wanted to know about the disease. Finally, she ended the date by saying I'm a nice guy, but … "I could never get romantically involved with you because of your sickness." I laughed and said I knew an hour ago and I felt badly for her because she was missing out on a great life. You can't change the whole world, all you can control is your response to what it throws at you. Sometimes you catch a rose, and sometimes you get hit with a brick. Be prepared and accepting of the rose, but remember that not every brick is your fault!

Dating and Acromegaly are not easy. Neither is marriage and Acromegaly. Over the course of my modern life, I have been honored to have many people confide in me about their own struggles with Acro. I think everyone's favorite topic is the relationship path. The human need for emotional support is huge, and very real. If I were to give any advice here based on my own experiences, as well as the stories I have been told, I would say that if you are married or in a serious relationship with someone traveling this path, love that person when they are least lovable—because that is when they need you the most. But if you are the patient in that same relationship, be sensitive to your lover. Generally speaking, we know when things are bad. Try to work to overcompensate when you feel low. If you can't, or you just have nothing left in the tank, you need to excuse yourself from their presence and try to get yourself composed. We have an emotionally charged disease, and it takes a team effort to make it function.

I know that a lot of people without any medical issues have a hard time managing personality conflicts in a relationship. Normal relationships are complicated! Patients, we have a duty to try our best when we feel our worst. But loved ones, sometimes we won't always succeed. Please understand that we are probably very aware of our demeanor, and we are struggling to screw on a smile. Yelling at us or demeaning us will not make it come about easier. If we love each other, and we choose to be with each other, then we both need to be sympathetic to these very real struggles.

Managing the Disease, Rather than the Disease Managing You

Sometimes having Acromegaly makes you feel like you have multiple personalities. I had so many mood swings with such randomness of emotion that I used to feel like I was going crazy, not to mention what I did to the people around me. Most of the other patients I have talked with about anger know the feeling of having regular bad moods and then their Acro-anger. While this usually improves when medically treated and controlled, bad days still happen, and there is little predicting when that little Acro-monster will pop his head up and ruin your moment, your event, or your whole day. While it can be difficult, we still have the responsibility to manage our own issues; *especially when we feel it coming on.* It is in your best interest to get to know yourself so you can best control your issues, causing as little stress for other people as possible. I know that when my profession brings stress about, I can have a visit from my little Acro-monster, so I need to be sensitive to thinking before I speak. Acro-monster seems to like to pop up when I am hyper-extended in responsibilities, tasks, or stress; but one sarcastic comment made in frustration can forever change a relationship with another person.

One of the best things a patient can do for themselves is to really and truly get to know themselves. While this may seem obvious or self-aggrandizing to people on the surface, getting to truly understand yourself can be one of life's most difficult tasks. It takes a great deal of uncomfortable honestly and self-criticism. My earliest memories involve my parents encouraging my creativity; and my gift was communication, my method: humor. I love to make people laugh because I love when people are happy. My earliest exposure to stand-up comedy was when my cousin was babysitting me and my sister. Soon after we went to bed one night, she came and got me because there was a show on cable she really wanted me to see: *George Carlin: Carlin on Campus.* It was love at first sight! From then on, while my friends were buying music cassettes, I was buying George Carlin, Eddie Murphy, and Richard Pryor albums. Brilliant comedians, and my parents figured that I really didn't *understand* why the jokes were so funny (in hindsight, they were probably right). When I was healthy, all was fine. Occasionally I told a joke that made mom and dad cringe, but that was it. As I got older though, and my pituitary betrayed me, I had an inventory of inappropriate humor trapped in my brain. It is amazing just how quickly a person can lose friends when they are always trying to be funny, but it comes out as mean.

I finally made a deal with myself to try to improve how people saw me. I had friends, but they were not all people that made me happy. Many of the good people in my life hung out with me out of obligation or habit, but they knew that it was likely I would have some sort of fit during the course of an evening. It is not that my anger was always unjustified, but the level of anger was not always appropriate for the situation. After I started getting treated for the Acromegaly, I quickly became aware of how many people in my life, including family, feared my mood swings. I was at a crossroads. I could either blame the people because they did not understand me or I could say that it was my fault.

I used to have a favorite phrase when I would try to help someone understand a shortcoming with themselves that everyone else saw. This was the idea that "everybody else can't be wrong." Finally, one day it hit me that I was just as blind as the people I tried to offer advice to. When I finally faced that knowledge, I needed to figure out what was causing my problems so I could figure out how to fix my issues. As I saw it, I needed to commit myself to improving my attitude. This did not mean immediately running up to people and apologizing for years of poor behavior; it simply meant I needed to change how I thought, and how I communicated what I thought. *Rule number one for me from me was to think before I spoke.* If there was any doubt about it, SHUT UP! I knew that it would take a while for people to see the change in me, but it was a change worthwhile. As if Hollywood was speaking to me, I was watching a movie one night around my epiphany, and the moral of the movie story was that a person can undergo a major life transformation, even in their 30s. Towards the end of the movie when the guy is at his high school reunion, an old friend asked how his life was. He simply responded, "In progress." *Wow! If this guy can change his entire life so dramatically, so can I!* I knew somewhere in the back of my mind that it was just a movie, but that didn't matter. I decided that I was going to fix my negative attitude, and when I set my mind to a mission, it is going to happen.

I started out just by making a conscious effort to have a smile on my face, rather than a scowl. Also, I kept mind of my jokes before I said them. I decided that while I like being the funniest person in the room, I knew the look of pain on the person I had just humiliated with a joke I thought was harmless. The goal was to blend in, rather than be the focal point of an event. The problem was that I really did not know how to blend. After so many years of being known as "big guy," I still didn't know how to respond to the pain that comment caused. My response could go one of two ways: either I would internalize the pain or make an obnoxious comment in reply. I finally realized there was another option. Smile and let it go, until I could talk to the other person in private. Generally speaking, people are reasonable about fixing their missteps!

I thought that it was going to take forever for people to notice the attitude change, but people perceived the change in my personality quite quickly. Far more quickly than I would have ever imagined. One day, only a couple months after I started trying to change the Wayne I presented to the rest of the world, I overheard someone say, "What happened to Wayne? He was really a lot of fun to be around today!" I knew that this was a kind of backward compliment, but I needed to take the compliment part and just build on the feedback. This would be my life for a little while: take the compliment, no matter how much it may sting. Luckily, it did not take too long for people to grow accustomed to my new personality, especially when the changes were so positive.

As the years have moved along since discovering that I had to work on my attitude, I have noticed a definite change in the people I surround myself with and how we see each other. It is a constant battle that I need to be wary of, and I need to always be vigilant of the person that others are seeing. When I get stressed, it is easier to lose control than keep quiet; but I have to make sure I make good choices.

I was in a work setting during a recent winter where I was coming into the building with my satchel, my laptop computer, my lunch bag, and my coffee thermos. I was wearing a heavy goose down coat, carrying my mail from the main office after signing in, and thinking about the work to come that day. All I had left was to unlock my door and disassemble this mess—an easy enough task for an octopus but not so much for a human being. Sitting in the hallway watching me struggle was the hall monitor wishing me an extremely sing-songy good morning. Now the old Wayne would have launched a tirade as to why she was so stupid as to either not help me or to wait until I was more settled. While my getting upset at this lady may have made me feel better for a brief moment, it was not going to help our relationship at all; and what would happen when I saw her tomorrow, and tomorrow, and tomorrow? One second's catharsis could result in several months of ill will. Overtaxed, I saw the white light and knew what little monster was perched on my shoulder. Whenever I want to have an Acro-spaz, it is usually preceded with an anger that is so passionate that I can actually see white; and not just any white, it is a white light like you would see by staring at a noontime sun during the summer. Rather than giving in, I just self-talked myself down. "Wayne, just say good morning and shut up!" I take orders from myself on issues of anger pretty well, so that is what I did. I grumbled a *mornin'* and then disappeared into my classroom. I set everything down and felt the anger wash away. I could literally see and feel the white light just wash away. Now I am relieved that I kept my mouth under control because nothing ever happened, no one felt bad or awkward, and no apologies were needed. I grabbed my coffee cup and sighed a deep sigh. I gave myself a mental pat on the back for doing what I knew was right, in spite of how I felt, and walked out of the classroom.

Now I gave the lady a genuine and *warm* good morning. The day would go on as if nothing had happened because it didn't. And the fact that nothing happened was due, in large part, to my getting to know myself and working around my shortcomings. This would actually end up becoming part of my morning work routine. I don't know why she never got the hint that I was happier after I put everything away, but so be it; I also don't know why I would still feel the anger, knowing what the morning dialogue was going to be even before getting to work.

Tips from a Patient on How I Manage My Acro-Anger

Stories like the above could fill the next thousand pages. I am sure that all the patients reading this story could add a million of their own stories as well. As patients with Acromegaly, we need to be very aware of our emotional stability. We need to remember that we have a rare disease, and that means that almost everybody we know will not relate to our bad days. I have learned an awful lot on emotional management from the common housecat. No matter how badly a cat is hurt, it never lets you see it in pain.

One of my defense mechanisms is the seeking of close friends. I have a very select group of people I feel I can talk to with total honesty. This is not easy. Be careful of who you say what to. If they are not acromegalic, no matter how much they love you, sympathy will not always be there. One comment in the heat of emotion can never be unheard or unsaid. I remember that soon after I was diagnosed with Acromegaly, I was talking with someone and they asked how I was doing. Foolishly, I answered honestly. I said I just felt lousy. Their response was that I always complain. I am still close with that person, but I am always aware of what I talk about with them.

Sometimes a momentary comment in the heat of frustration can cause an irreparable rift though. When Michelle and I were having a lot of disagreements, towards the end of the relationship, I was fighting to keep it together. Then she said in the heat of an argument that had nothing to do with my disease, "You always blame the stupid disease for everything." That was the moment I broke my emotional bond with her. We were done. I did not say anything, but I just lost the desire to care for her. That was the second I had fallen totally out of love with her, and we have never talked since that conversation. She has reached out since then, but I don't want to let her back in. People can be ignorant because they are ignorant of what we deal with: big guy, banana hands, Frankenstein, etc. I am pretty sure I have heard them all. They are not all meant as insults, sometimes they are meant as terms of endearment. But when a patient is overly aware of their physical appearance, a person's nickname can cut very deeply.

The best advice I can give a patient is to know who you can speak with. Be wary of those you trust. If you need someone to talk with that is not emotionally connected to you, invest in a psychologist or counselor. Make sure they are a good fit though. Just because someone has a good reputation does not mean he/she is a good fit for you. I used to be very good at cocooning myself when I was having a particularly bad day, but luckily that is only one option now. Yes, there are days when I just need to hide from the world. As an acromegalic, you must be patient with yourself and accept the fact that sometimes this is just necessary. If you feel lousy and you don't want to talk, you have that right. If you do want to talk with people though, there are options.

Patients Supporting Each Other- A Community Is Born

I would have to imagine that navigating a disease when you are surrounded by people who can understand your pain and your challenges is still difficult, but doing it totally by yourself can be positively excruciating. Most acromegalics will go through their entire lives without ever meeting another person with the same aches, pains, concerns, and questions; so it is up to us to manage ourselves. If you are lucky enough to meet another patient, this is a huge help in curing the feelings of isolation.

I will always remember the first time I met other acromegalics for the first time. It was in March of 2009. For the first time since my diagnosis I was able to shake hands and hug and share stories with people who would say "me too" instead of looking at me either with pity, contempt, or disbelief. Empathy can be an amazing catharsis when you have spent years of your life trapped in your own misery because you did not want to be the wet blanket of the crowd, and explaining yourself feels like it takes too long.

The best people ultimately to talk with are people affected by the disease. The internet is a wonderful avenue for meeting people with specialized issues. One night I was sitting home alone, mired in my solitude. I decided to create a group on MySpace for people with Acromegaly, just to see if I could meet some other patients. A few people joined, but not many. All the same, I still got to chat with other Acromegalics. The world felt a lot less lonely. In 2007 I joined Facebook, and the first thing I did was to create a new Acromegaly Support group. Again, it grew slowly, but I met even more new people. As the years have passed, more people have joined our family. Not just patients, but friends and family of patients too. What happens here is absolutely fantastic. People share stories, jokes, frustrations, fears, ideas, and SUPPORT. While I love the family that nature gave me, there is a part of my life that they are lucky enough to really not have any access to. I had a local news station do a feature about me, and it amazed me how many people who I am close to said "I didn't know that ..." Meanwhile, my Acro family saw the piece and said, "Thank you for sharing our reality with the rest of the world." I love my natural family, but when I am having a bad day, I can't live without my Acro family. We now have these social networking sites to use. They are invaluable. In addition, we have a message board on AcromegalyCommunity.com that is open to patients and their loved ones, conference calls of support, and even a newsletter. The key focus we have is to make sure that people who feel alone have someone to reach out to.

We orphan disease patients are enjoying the beginning of a kind of renaissance. We have options on how to get to know each other. If you need to hide, you can. But if you want to come out and join the rest of us, there are many wonderful people around the globe who would love to talk with you and support you.

The future is upon us. If you are a patient, a loved one, or a friend, join us. AcromegalyCommunity is about mutual support. We are all at different points on our journey, and we would love to have you share your experiences.

Wayne Brown, M. Ed., is the founder of Acromegaly Community, Inc. As a former High School Social Studies teacher, he became quite skilled at leading and inspiring by example. He earned his Master of Education from State University College at Buffalo. Wayne has been featured in *The New York Times*' "Patient Voices" for his experiences with Acromegaly. He has also been published in the *Washington Post*, *Wall Street Journal*, and *Buffalo News*.

Looking through the Window: Acromegaly as Seen by a Friend Wayne . . . Before and After

Ray Graf

"I believe that if life gives you lemons, you should make lemonade... And try to find somebody whose life has given them vodka, and have a party."

—Ron White

A Future Friend on First Sight

The man I befriended before 2000 was not the man I knew after that date. Being asked to describe the "real Wayne" back then might be even tougher than it is now. When we met, that first sighting reminded me of a local car commercial where an oversized promoter just yells "HUUUGE" into the camera at the end of the ad.

Once you got to know Wayne, you could see that the biggest part of his body was his heart. But until you got to know him, you couldn't help but notice that Wayne was really big in general. Even his personality was huge. When Wayne walked into a room, he filled it in every way. His laugh could stifle conversations, his hands could sweep cups of drinks onto laps, and his wit could suppress any comeback. That being said, he didn't really laugh a whole lot. The dropping of drinks usually came with a frustrated grunt, and the wit came with a sarcastic and sometimes biting comment.

As everyone including Wayne would later find out, he was dealing with Acromegaly, and his features were actually quite typical for people with that disease. His condition was in no way helped by living in Buffalo, New York, a place known to be a "drinking town with a football problem." With homemade ethnic food on every corner, micro-brewed beers all over the place, greasy food that goes well with many losing sports teams, and the ever-famous chicken wings, I'm sure this compounded what would have made a challenging condition all but impossible to manage.

Meeting Wayne in college was interesting. We were both students in a small school with an even smaller History & Government department. Wayne and I started out as almost total opposites in every way. I was a college cross-country runner who was never very good but loved to try to improve—at our school that made me a wanna-be jock. I was very self-conscious about my weight and had a lack of athletic prowess, so I worked through my physical issues and joined the Marine Corps Reserves. I also started out as a Graphic Design major but realized that a B+ in art would probably lead me to "B" standing in the unemployment line, so I switched over to History & Government and decided to try and become a teacher. I was inspired by a few of our professors, and the next thing I knew, I was writing my own Presidential Journal so that when I became president after finishing with undergrad and the Reserves, I would already have the habit down. My idealism about how easy it would be to change society and fight for what was right in a clear, polite manner came naturally. (No, I was not as bad as Hank Hill from TV's *King of the Hill*, but it was close.) This stood in direct contrast to Wayne and was spelled out perfectly during one of our first meetings.

It was the infamous 2000 election where George W. Bush and Al Gore went toe-to-toe, and the History & Government department at our college was throwing a party to watch the returns, foolishly thinking the election could be decided in one night. I was there and, along with almost everyone else at our small, liberal college party, was thinking, "How could anyone possibly vote Republican in this election?" Wayne was there, and I could already tell he did not fit the mold when he began arguing with one of our professors about how Bush would win and the Democrats were backing a loser. What was more remarkable to me was that Wayne was arguing with a man who had aided students in protesting the Vietnam War, and he was in no way dissuaded in his passion or his argument. I don't know if any of us believed him, but after a mere thirty-six days of vote-counting, W was declared the winner. All I could think about was my Reserve contract: "I have five more years left on my contract and I can't even speak out against my Commander-in-Chief." For Wayne and me, that meeting at that party served to set up a benchmark for the next so many years of our time in college.

Our collegiate relationship became a very clear, persistent love-hate relationship. We both had very distinct and opposing ideas on politics and current events, but more than that, we were both very vocal about our perspectives. Because we were both history geeks with a penchant for pre-law studies, arguing was in our nature. Always good-natured, and usually well-conducted, we became sounding boards for each other to bounce ideas off of—frequently at a very loud pitch. I took a liberal view; his was conservative. It seemed to everyone walking past the lounge where we ate cookies, drank coffee, and debated with anyone who would listen, that we hated each other when in fact, we were great friends.

A second difference, Wayne espoused the philosophy of "Life sucks, deal with it." As previously mentioned, I was going to fix the world (I still can—we just need democratic-totalitarianism—you elect me and I will do all of your thinking for you); he was cynical about the world even being able to be fixed. I tried to argue a kinder, more sympathetic, "Things shouldn't be the way they are, let's tweak this just a bit." Wayne was much more pessimistic: "This is the way the world is, adapt to it and quit complaining."

Another obvious and unavoidable contrast between Wayne and me was inevitably plain and simple: he was older. On a campus where most people were worried about finding ways to get alcohol, going to Canada to party, and getting their nighttime drivers' licenses so they could drive after 9:00 p.m., Wayne had other cares. He had an accountant and was concerned about his mortgage, his health care, and most importantly, his insurance rates. Our friends sometimes played a game with Wayne: "Was I born when Wayne . . .," and this might have been followed up with "saw Frampton in concert," "watched the Bills play in a Super Bowl," or (my favorite) "graduated from high school." Wayne did a very good job adapting as best he could, but whereas I was getting my first checking account that didn't have my mother listed as "guardian," he had already run his own business. Most of the students were living in dorms without cars, but Wayne owned his own house and had a fancy car, two dogs, and multiple jobs to maintain it all. It was like we had two totally different existences.

There were some other "non-traditional" students in the group whom Wayne easily connected with, and he regularly encouraged them to join in our circle and socialize. I think it was nice for them to be able to talk about things like "remember when cell phones were connected to a briefcase?" It wasn't like he couldn't relate to people of all ages; he did connect well, and helped many others to join our group. But ultimately, most of the kids in our college group were "wet behind the ears." He, on the other hand, had *extensive* life experience before attending college *this* time. Always one to have thick skin, Wayne could joke about the number of previous college attempts. And before he returned to college, he had owned his own business (somewhat successfully, but ultimately not), had done stand-up comedy, and (before and during college) had written articles for local and national newspapers. He had an extensive knowledge of sports, especially hockey. One of the most life-changing events that affected him was a somewhat-critical car accident that forced him to constantly work through medications and treatments that ultimately narrowed his career choices and job opportunities. I know he was struggling to figure out his path in college, initially thinking of law school, until one night he called me from work to ask about the education program. He asked a bunch of questions until he eventually believed it was something he could do, and wanted to try. His love of history, and ultimately his love of helping children, streamlined him into the same Social Studies Education Program as me, and that is where we would finally cross paths.

It was no wonder that when Wayne threw himself into this kind of environment, with one of even his close friends in the program being so different, he might not feel totally comfortable all the time in that atmosphere. Wayne's discomfort might have been at least partially compounded by Wayne's own personality though.

At the time, Wayne's personality could be defined by one word: sarcasm. Though I've never seen his stand-up comedy act, based on what I know of him, I would have to assume that he was an insult comic. Don't get me wrong, he was never demeaning or hurtful, but his comments were always biting. There was a core group of mutual friends who became close and constantly hung out during this college time. The group loved him, but often we were slower to speak in his presence, unsure if our comment would lead to a biting retort that we would have to counter. Wayne was funny, but he wasn't always fun. The ironic part was that even when he would have fun, he often didn't seem to enjoy it. It was as if he was mad at life and even his occasional happiness was mocking him. No matter how happy he was, he seemed to always feel that he had to be ready for a cruel "second shoe" to drop. There is an episode of a famous cartoon comedy series in which the wise cafeteria advisor says something like "God gives us happiness so that when he takes it away, things hurt that much more. It's your tears that make God happy." It almost seemed that every time Wayne was happy, he braced for the sadness to follow.

I think that his unhappiness stemmed from the constant battles he was forced to fight to kind of "get through life." Working crummy jobs of long hours that started before school and continued after school, writing papers, then coming into classes in between would drain almost anyone. Wayne struggled with student-teaching, working, lesson planning, spending time with friends, and fitting in sleep whenever he could. Wayne always seemed to adapt, but looking back on the experiences now, it seems that the longer I knew him, the more things got to him. The cynicism seemed to get pretty bad when he got more tired and closer to graduation. We all had similar experiences and they all weighed on everybody heavily; but given the list of extra obstacles Wayne was dealing with, I can't imagine anyone expecting him not to get at least a little frustrated.

One of the most trying, and telling, experiences I saw was when we went on a History & Government department trip to Washington, DC. The trip was an experience that we've talked about for years. We drove down from Western New York in a college van. In the van were two single ladies, a dating couple, our college professor, and Wayne and I, also both single. Needless to say, it was a very diverse group with very few numbers to be diverse with. On the way down, I got a speeding ticket. When we got to the halfway point, one member of our party decided it would be a better idea to change all the previous travel arrangements and switch hotels. The new hotel would be a shorter drive, but it put us in a rougher part of town. It was also at this point that Wayne took over and navigated through the crowded and congested parts to find us the new hotel, and eventually we started doing the tourist things.

The main purpose of the trip was to see the Holocaust Museum. The Museum was very well done but, as any history nerd will tell you, "well done" means "cool" but not to everybody in every context. There were some members of our party who thought it would also be "cool" to take pictures at certain points of the Museum, some of them inappropriate. This bothered Wayne a bit, but he took it in stride as the cultural impact of events affects everybody differently. His patience did not last forever; dealing with the many different personalities grated on his nerves more than the rest of us, and he was the first to get really frustrated. When the group wanted to travel to Georgetown, but then found out how expensive the bars were, Wayne was the first to get ticked. When the group thought the zoo would be fun, Wayne was the one who (justifiably) said, "Uh, there are zoos everywhere. Why are we going to one on our trip, now?" He went along with it though he let it eat away at him, and he stewed about it until we were leaving the exit after seeing all the lions, tigers, and bears. A few beers at the hotel bar eventually smoothed things over a bit, but whereas the rest of the group was annoyed but had fun, it seemed like Wayne was actually really ticked. There seemed to be little about the trip that he thought was worthwhile, and I really thought that he thought that many of the people were not even decent human beings. After conversing with him, though, I found out that while Wayne was annoyed and did think the trip might have been better, he actually thought the people we went with were fine. Apparently he was only unhappy at the specific time even though I thought at times that he might have slaughtered the lot of us. I would never have guessed without the conversation that he had fun. Just by his physical appearance, the way his shoulders slumped, the scowl, the shamble to his walk, all eked "You people are ticking the crap out of me." Instead of finding something nice about the experience, he seemed miserable on the surface.

With Wayne, we also saw this annoyance outside of the college environment. When we would go out to dinner, he was often abrupt with the wait staff. His complaints were often valid, but he would sometimes allow a trivial slight to offend and disrupt his dining experience. At times, it was a fear among our group that something negative might happen. It was not because we were concerned about our experience but because we were concerned Wayne might have a conflict that would then affect the dynamic of the whole group. There were really not that many trying experiences, but when there were, it made things sometimes uncomfortable, especially for someone who tends to be an overly polite "no, ma'am, I wanted my fries cold, but since you asked, I really wouldn't mind your reheating them" boy. In one very minor case, the waitress started bringing our food, and because there were at least five or six people in the party, by the time she got around to dropping off all the plates and getting our drinks, she asked us how everything was before we'd had a chance to eat anything. This inspired Wayne to tell her that he hadn't eaten anything yet, and after he actually had tasted it, he would let her know. The rest of us told her things looked fine, but it did inspire a few minutes of conversation about how one should ask about the quality of food and when. Though the waitress was never really offended, it gave a quick peek into Wayne seeing the negative instead of the positive.

There are just as many intangible examples of experiences where things just didn't seem right but almost always had justifiable excuses. At our college, part of our senior thesis project was to present our findings at the school's annual Academic Festival. In each session, three speakers were given a block of time to present in, with each person getting an equal part and turning the presentation over to the next speaker. Anyone who wanted to attend was invited, and when each presentation was completed, the audience could ask questions. The man before Wayne ended up taking a good ten to fifteen minutes more than his allotted time, justifiably ticking off Wayne and much of the audience. It wasn't that he was vocal about his anger; it was that the way he showed it seemed to take over his whole body. His presentation was efficient and interesting, and he adapted well; but there was the underlying feeling that he had been slighted. This was not unusual when something presented a challenge for Wayne. When we were taking our teacher certification tests, we had to complete one test in the morning and then another in the afternoon; each one cost about $100 (which neither of us really had), and if we failed, we would have to keep retaking them until we passed. By the end of the first, we were both "done" but met during lunch to take a break before going back for the afternoon. I felt tired, but it seemed that all Wayne's strength was gone and that he was just beat down. As a happy ending to this story, we both passed all our tests on the first try.

Wayne participated in many school activities. He always participated in class discussions and really enjoyed being in the academic arena. He got great grades, but seemed to have to work harder than his peers just to do comparatively well. Wayne became a natural leader who did not seem to necessarily enjoy being the center of attention. Some of our friends strove to become leaders on campus. They would struggle and work at becoming club president or committee chairperson. Wayne didn't try but when asked would always step up. Serving as a lead proctor at a county-wide High School Model United Nations, becoming president of the History & Government Club, or acting in a play on campus, Wayne was always there to help. In some cases he was asked to take over and be in charge, in others it was to coordinate or accomplish a portion of a task.

Wayne's style of leadership was efficient but in some cases viewed as kind of dictatorial. The best example may be the way he used to give advice. As someone who was alive to see Reagan speak and who might have actually voted for both Bushes, experiencing what he did, his advice did come with some clout, but with little sympathy; and while his advice was usually good, it was often not a suggestion. "But of course that's what you should do . . . it's not arguing, just do it." Wayne often didn't give the option of discussing the advice; if it was right, it was right. I still remember sitting in the lounge trying to argue the merits of another choice for an event we were planning and

Wayne just saying something like, "Yeah, okay, but this is better. No. This is better. Stop thinking about it. This is better. Just do this."

One major hypothesis as to why Wayne was Wayne among our friends was simply that he was big. On top of that, while many of his friends were athletic, Wayne was out of shape. After the car accident, he had been struggling with his weight, and it went up and down on a regular basis. He always had a large frame and would be considered "solid" to look at by almost any passive observer. It wasn't so much that he had no athletic ability; in fact he was very strong. It just seemed that he never had the coordination to move well, and that kind of made any extra weight he was carrying sit heavy on him.

Personally, I consider myself to be extremely lacking in coordination. I think I made up for it with running in a straight line so at least I looked like I knew what I was doing (but even still I managed to fall a few times a year). I saw many of the same coordination struggles in Wayne that I was dealing with, only his issues seemed so much more magnified. Sports that required finely tuned skills like volleyball or bowling were tough for Wayne to be elegant in. Whereas I would hit the volleyball and it would fly into the net, or in the opposite direction of the net, Wayne might hit the ball into a neighboring building. When it came to bowling, he could literally throw the ball halfway down the alley before it hit the floor. In one crazy example, I was so impressed I rolled three strikes in the last frame (making my score a great 147 for me). I didn't think Wayne could do much against me, and I was hurting my shoulder to pat myself on the back so much. Lo and behold, his ball actually rolled down, went into the gutter, bounced out, and took down two or three pins in the final frame. I stopped patting and shook his hand. These coordination issues we assumed were from his bad back from the car accident. It was all the injury, not anything else. And we certainly did not think it was because of a tumor!

His physical aspects were not all negative. As a workout partner, he was no slouch with the weights, and with the help of cardio exercises, he began to lose some weight. When we went to the gym (there were three of us), Wayne was by far the largest of the three. After we finished a solid workout, I would go to shower and change, and Wayne and our mutual friend would bolt outside for a cigarette.

After I finished showering and they finished smoking, Wayne and I would indulge our mutual friend's penchant for fast-food buffet restaurants. While this did not help any of our physiques, with the amount of exercises we were all doing, we all got stronger; and Wayne seemed to show the greatest strength gains without losing a whole lot of weight. Even allowing for the bad food choices, this was definitely one very clear sign among many that something just didn't seem right. Even as he got stronger and more defined, his overall weight did not seem to diminish; especially in areas like his face and neck, the weight loss was never noticeable. His stomach would trim and his arms and legs would get muscular, but that seemed to be about it.

But the gym was not the only unusual aspect of Wayne's issues. His consumption of coffee was like nothing I had ever seen before. He would carry an extra-large cup, almost the size of an iced tea pitcher, and polish it off repeatedly during a day. When it came to consumption of food, drink, or anything else he enjoyed, quantity was never an issue. Though he did not drink alcohol on a nightly basis, he could easily consume many more drinks than his peers. Our workout buddy teased that we should have a drinking contest, Wayne against the two of us. With me being such an alcohol "lightweight" and Wayne seeming to be able to put away so much more than me, it might have been interesting. I *could* put away a whole pizza by myself even then, and Wayne was right with me in terms of food quantity. It wasn't just what he ate, it was how. When eating, rather than pick up one french fry at a time, he would grab clumps of three or four fries and eat them as one. He didn't have an insatiable urge to pound down fries, but I'm not sure he had the patience/coordination to try something with such fine motor coordination. He was not a pig, but he was not a patient eater. And while I am not heavy, I have a big appetite that few people can keep up with, so if someone can match my eating, they can put away the food. (Side note: Many people think that because I ran and still do run "so much" that I am very healthy with what I eat. In fact, I run so much because I eat so much.)

Wayne had a lot of issues, and all of his friends knew that. With severe back pain at times, the loss of his father at a young age, health issues with his mother and grandmother (both of whom were lovely, kind, and doting women), the loss of a career, his hefty size, trying to get through school a second time with others who were much younger that he, and the lack of a religious crutch, none of us could blame him for feeling disgruntled. We certainly did not think that we were seeing warning signs that something medically serious might exist, other than the results of the car accident. We just always assumed that this was "just Wayne," and we accepted him for what he was. After all, that is what friends are supposed to do, right?

Then the Wayne we all knew died . . . metaphorically. . .

Mr. Hyde and Dr. FeelBetter?

Wayne didn't die in the physical sense, obviously. But when he discovered that he needed to have, for all intents and purposes, brain surgery, we were all shocked. At first, our friends would talk, saying thoughts like "how much more could this guy get screwed by the world?" It seemed that something bad was always happening to him. He spent so much of his time managing health issues with his family members and doing volunteer work at agencies where he dealt with tragedy, and all of this seemed to weigh on him enough already. Some of the stories he would tell were heartbreaking; others were just about people struggling with bad times. The health of his family was always a concern, but it was the way other stuff seemed to just drain him that really made us empathize with him. With all the living he did, he still seemed like he was just dealing with life. I just thought that he didn't seem like the kind of person with a brain tumor, although in hindsight, I am not sure what that person should look like.

The first portion of this chapter might have seemed to be harsh or maybe even hurtful. It is not intended this way, but I thought it was necessary to be totally honest. That way you could appreciate the extreme contrast that needs to be shown. Wayne today is a very different person than he was the day before his treatment started. I changed that last line because I initially wrote "totally" different person. Wayne is not totally different—the same guy I was friends with is still there, but it seems that he has become the person he wanted to be.

This is not to say that stress had left his life. Before the surgery, Wayne was on a pharmaceutical-maintenance program that seemed to be offering a lot of help; but it was not cheap. For some people, the idea of having a medication where you could die if you don't take it is incomprehensible, but to Wayne, it was a relief! One day, a few weeks after he started on his first-ever injections that he needed to administer three times a day, he was preparing the shot when he lost his coordination over the tiny glass vial, and it dropped to the ground, shattering. That same day I was hosting a small get-together at the house I was renting. While I had heard from Wayne only days before how much different he was feeling with this drug, when he walked in, you could just see in his eyes that things were not good. When I heard what happened, I couldn't fathom it. The idea that your life-saving, thousand-dollar medication was now shattered on the ground would be enough to wreck anyone's weekend. Wayne was still able to get through it. At some point—and I'm not sure I could have done it in the same situation—he was able to simply continue with life. Being away from the rest of life for a weekend may have helped, especially with a wise-cracking group of friends.

One benefit to Wayne's lifetime of wisdom was that he understood the importance of maintaining health coverage. Without health insurance, his medical maintenance would have been, at best, price prohibitive. More realistically, it would have bankrupted him. But thankfully he was always conscious of his need for continuous health insurance, and he has worked through very unpleasant situations to be able to stay insured. It has served as an example to me to keep things in order in case anything unexpected should ever happen to me. His persistence paid off, and when it was time for his surgery, I could never have imagined the difference.

I actually went to see him the day after his release from the hospital. He had a caretaker helping him around the house, and physically, he looked no different than before. But when I sat down with him at the table, the difference became immediately apparent. Though physically exhausted from the surgery, I had never heard him so emotionally relieved. Neither he nor I could believe the way he was feeling. Though the exact comments escape my memory, I remember him saying something to the effect of "I never knew how bad I felt before until now." He couldn't stop talking about how much better he felt. Eventually he began nodding off during our conversation, and I took my leave for the evening. But the emotion was apparent: "You cannot believe how much better I feel."

As time has passed over the years since surgery, Wayne's complaints about his pain, both back and otherwise, have diminished. His disposition has become amazingly better. Instead of biting sarcasm when problems arise, he laughs. When he got a hernia from too much weightlifting and actually needed surgery again, he was the one laughing about how dumb he was to put himself in that situation. Even through the aches and pain, holding his stomach, he didn't stop smiling and laughing. Instead of being frustrated by these parts of his life that were not going well, we joked about it.

Now when we go out to restaurants, both his diet and his whole demeanor have changed. Going out for dinner has become a treat. Wayne used to communicate simply: "Give me the blank." After the surgery, things were fun. Wayne's voice changed to the "telephone voice" of sweetness and sincerity whenever communicating with the wait staff. When there was confusion, instead of being mad and angry or getting almost snotty with the staff, he would laugh it off. A classic example was when a bunch of our close friends went out for Thai food. The waitress was taking our order when this exchange took place:

Waitress: How would like your dish?
Ray: I need it very mild please, no spice.
Waitress: Thank you. And you sir?
Wayne: I'll have the Pru Wan.
Waitress: And how would you like it?
Wayne: I'll have it like, warm.
Waitress: Uhm, all our dishes are served cooked.
Wayne: No, I mean not hot, but warm.
Waitress: Uh yes, if it is too hot, it can cool down…
Wayne: No like medium hot/spicy.
Waitress: Oh, okay.

Before diagnosis and treatment, there would have been a concern about Wayne getting mad at the staff. Now, we almost split our sides laughing in hysterics. If Wayne was embarrassed or bothered by the exchange, no one would have known because even Wayne was shaking his head and snickering. It was a classic example of the new Wayne.

Wayne has become better at managing life's occasional wrinkles. Being history geeks, when an exhibit on Catherine the Great came to Toronto from the Hermitage, Wayne and I *had to* go. Even though the ride was long and it was cold during this Christmas break from school, it seemed nothing could bother him. I was a bit nervous about making the poor guy drive the whole way, but he had a GPS and seemed okay with driving. I hoped he would have fun. Even though there were the usual problems with travelling and crowds, he was the one taking everything in stride; it was me that was overly concerned. I think the comment he said most throughout the course of the night was *relax*. I think I was shocked that he was so cool about everything, even when things didn't work well, and it really impressed me.

Managing his pharmaceutical life has had an impact on Wayne's social life. A few months after he had surgery, Wayne was starting to feel symptoms return, and he needed to get back on medication. This time, the doctor wanted him to take a shot that only needed to be given once every four weeks. Unfortunately the doctor was unaware of how the shot would react with his body, and the aftereffects of the shot were awful. Wayne would refer to "shot weekend," and we all knew that he would need to take at least a full day of rest after each shot was administered; sometimes he would need to take off the whole weekend. In some cases, this totally changed our plans, and we just expected Wayne to come if or when he could. The last thing we wanted was to hear about Wayne falling asleep or passing out while driving. We all learned to work around the medication, but even this changed over time.

After about two years of Wayne taking the shot that he really didn't like but understood was vital to his good health, he got the opportunity to try a new prescription. While the "unknown" of a new drug was somewhat scary, it was still being tested by the FDA, so he would get it free for six months. With his job future in limbo at the time, it was a worthwhile decision. Wayne immediately felt a difference with the new medication, and he is now fully functional after taking the injection. Most recently, I have noticed that even on "shot days," we have been able to go out to eat immediately following the injection with no adverse effects. "I won't be around because I have to take my shot" has now turned into, "I should be okay, but I have to take my shot that weekend." I even got the chance to show my camera skills when Wayne demonstrated his injection routine for a web-based video. Not only was he able to take the injection in front of the camera in one take, we got dinner afterwards from a place we walked to.

Amazingly, Wayne has continued in a drive to improve his life, and he has definitely changed over time. Not only has he felt good enough to get back in the gym, he has been eating healthy and shedding weight like it was his job. With this, his features are shrinking at an alarming rate. His overall weight loss is extreme, but what is really noteworthy is the difference in things like his glove size. Even his face seems to have changed. He still has his "hero chin," but even that is smaller. He is still large enough to be imposing in any scuffle, but is now much more confident, healthy, and happy.

Before the surgery and shots, Wayne and I substitute taught at the same high school. Wayne taught for a teacher on one day, and I taught for the same teacher on the very next day. The kids told me about the sub they'd had the day before: "Yeah, you're totally different than the guy we had last time. He was this huge Italian-looking guy with these huge hands. I would not want to get on that guy's bad side." It wasn't what he said, how he said it, or what he taught that the kids remembered. Nothing was remembered except his size. This is not to say Wayne was a bad teacher; in fact, the opposite is true. It is important that his size was so imposing; that is what stood out in these kids' minds. In contrast, after the surgery, Wayne was a significant part of my wedding. During the ceremony, he sang a duet, led a toast, and was in many different photos. Instead of standing out in the black suit of the wedding party because of his size, he stood out by being himself. He received comments from a number of people who remarked on how well he spoke, how funny he was, and how confident he was. Even my mother noticed the change in how dynamic he was. Nobody ever mentioned his size. It was a key benchmark in an amazing transformation.

Though Wayne has physically developed into a size that fits him better, the biggest surprise to me and all his friends are the emotional differences. It seems that every pound he has shed has removed another chunk of negativity from his personality. Wayne seems to enjoy feeling good. His disposition is amazing. The best part of talking to Wayne used to be making him laugh because it didn't happen all that often. Now he seldom stops smiling and laughing during a conversation. Still struggling to change society (that democratic-totalitarianism is *not* going well), I seem to be finding life more and more discouraging. It is Wayne who keeps me upbeat. Our friends now accuse me of being the negative one in the group, and Wayne's the happy one. Wayne now hosts parties and has tons of people of all ages entertained at the same time. Adjectives describing Wayne before were *cantankerous*, *grumpy*, and *sarcastic*. Now it seems that *pleasurable*, *fun*, and *enjoyable* are applied to him more often than not.

Wisdom for the Future

Anybody with a life-changing condition can learn from Wayne. Wayne has embraced his condition, and though it has not become what he sees himself as, he has turned his "lemons" into something much more fun and wants to help others do the same. He seems to have figured out the balancing act of having a life-changing condition without the life-changing condition ruling his life. All too often one portion of someone's life creeps into all others and affects their personality. They begin to see themselves as that portion of their personality instead of as the whole person. Sometimes it is a career (I can't do that; I'm a doctor) or a family relationship (No, my mother needs me this weekend). Wayne seems to be able to maintain a balance so that his medical condition is not what he sees in the mirror. Hopefully others can see the inspiration in this and apply it where they need the help.

In getting to know Wayne and being his friend, it wasn't like I had the option of saying "that's just Wayne's disease." I met Wayne before he was diagnosed, and we grew to know each other throughout the different phases of his discovering the disease. As we developed a better understanding, and after he was diagnosed and got his surgery, Wayne experienced some crazy changes in his life, influencing those of us around him. As a friend, my goal is always to support my friends in their trying moments. With Wayne, it tended to be pretty easy because it seemed that he did not want to dwell on things he couldn't control. Because he kept things as very matter-of-fact, it made it really easy to help him cope when things were tough. When he was with his friends, we were just his friends. Going to Dave and Buster's to play video games, jet boating on the Niagara River, or attending free concerts on the Niagara Gorge never turned into a whole evening about the tumor in his head. Going to history movies or just *Clerks II* didn't make a whole lot of connections to what Wayne was dealing with. He kept it out of a lot of our conversations, instead discussing other parts of "normal life." Though the tumor did come up occasionally, I hope his time with friends gave Wayne a break from dealing with the high-stress stuff he couldn't control much.

When our conversation did turn to treatments or the disease, I tried to be supportive and to listen to learn anything I could. I was not into doing research or trying to find some "new treatment" I could tell him about. I wasn't a doctor with any experience nor was I a therapist to help Wayne talk through any issues. At some point, advice, problem solving, suggestions—they didn't seem to make too much sense where a life-threatening disease was concerned. Wayne could see those experts, and I always assumed he didn't need that from me; he needed me to be his friend. I always tried to support him and focused instead on the other decisions and problems he was dealing with. I gave him more than my share of advice on car purchases, houses, professional complaints, relationships, and all those other things that, as a friend, I could comment on with some justifiable knowledge.

I think Wayne helped his friends a lot by being a good barometer of how he was feeling and what he wanted to talk about. By taking control of the process and managing his reactions and interactions with friends, I could help support him a bit better. When things started getting tough at times, Wayne and I knew how to distract each other. Sometimes it was simply a "Ray, I could really use dinner and a drink," and other times we would see the exhibits or reenactments that only a self-proclaimed "history geek" would find cool. By not changing for the disease, I think we adapted better.

As well as Wayne's doing, I can't help but think what might have been the case for him if he had known about the condition sooner and got the treatments that made him feel so much better. Would he still have appreciated the life he has now as much without the years of discomfort? I think he has moved beyond the past and is now concerned with helping as many other people as possible get the treatments they need so that they don't have to worry about any lost time.

Though it seems the lemons made him bitter to begin with, Wayne has found the vodka that has made his life fun. The challenge now is to see that there is enough vodka to go around. If there is the need for someone to toast to that, I know someone who can do a great job.

Ray Graf, M. Ed., is a successful teacher in a suburb of Buffalo, NY. He received his undergraduate degree in History & Government from Daemen College in Snyder, NY, which is where he met and became very close friends with Wayne Brown. Ray earned his Master's Degree in Creative Studies from Buffalo State College. In addition to his teaching, he is a very active competitive runner, and also coaches with the Silver Creek Black Knight Cross Country and Track Teams. Ray has been happily married since 2008 and has been an active volunteer with Acromegaly Community.

Women's Issues

Trena Mathis

Believe in your heart that something wonderful is about to happen.
—Author unknown

My name is Trena Mathis and this is my "Acro-story." I am a forty-seven-year-old college Air Traffic Control Instructor. I consider myself a very positive, direct person who is spiritual, but not necessarily religious. I have a wonderful, devoted, and caring husband whom I've had the great joy of being married to for over twenty-one years, and I am a mother to a beautiful, talented, super intelligent daughter who is just now entering college and has changed her major three times in the past month. We have all been through a challenging journey in this battle with Acromegaly. In this chapter, I would like to tell you about my experiences with the physical and emotional issues of Acromegaly from a woman's perspective, before, during, and after treatment. I hope it helps you with your journey.

Like most acromegalics I had been experiencing headaches, along with other seemingly unconnected maladies, for what I guess was twelve years before getting the correct diagnosis. I remember one of the first headaches hit me at work around 1996. It was so powerful that I knew it was not right. It felt like an ice pick was stuck into my head at the base of my skull and poking me in the back of my right eye. When describing it to friends and co-workers, they were quick to offer advice or diagnoses for the pain. One suggestion I most vividly remember was when someone asked me if I "recently started taking any new supplements or changed brands?" It made sense because I had just started taking a calcium supplement to ward off osteoporosis, and I chalked the headache up to that because it was new to my system. I took some Advil and it seemed to take care of it for the time. I continued taking Advil for a couple days, and the pain completely subsided.

I figured that that must have been it; my body was just adjusting to the change in supplements and that caused me to have headaches. So for the next few years, every time I had these chronic headaches, I would pass it off as a change of vitamin supplements or change in brand names that seemed to coincide with the pain. It seemed like every time these headaches came up, there was a change in supplements or brands, or I had PMS, or I was just stressed. There were and are differences in my "Acro-headaches" and ordinary ones. Normal headaches are all over or broad to me, whereas the "Acro-headache" is in one area at the base of the brain and penetrates to behind my right eye. I could feel it just behind where a swallowing motion starts in my throat. Later in the disease development, the pain also radiated to my right jawbone just below my ear. The "Acro-headache" for me was in a very specific place and easy to describe once I was given the opportunity.

Many of us can find reasons for our headaches and often don't take them seriously. We would rather medicate them and quickly make the pain go away rather than find the reason for it and fixing it permanently. Pain, especially when it's re-occurring, should always be an indicator that something serious could be going on. If I could tell the world this I would shout it—"PEOPLE, REOCCURRING HEADACHES ARE NOT NORMAL—GET IT CHECKED OUT—DEMAND AN MRI!!!!" I just hope that no one had a headache when I screamed that last line at you! If someone would have told me that back when mine first began, it could have saved me and my family from a lot of grief and suffering.

One of the causes I was given by medical professionals for my headaches was STRESS. In hindsight I am starting to wonder just how many times medical professionals glaze over serious issues and use this to explain things that their tests don't answer. Stress seems to be a bit of a catch-all to oversimplify a wide variety of physical symptoms and medical conditions. Too many times, a mother has too many of her symptoms blamed on the stress of being a new mother, being the mother of children under the age of five or being the mother of teenagers. I've heard it so many times that it is sickening. When I hear that "diagnosis," I want to shout, "Hell yes, I have stress and I am having a hard time with it. But I know my body, and this is more than just stress. Help me find a way to fix it!!" I was told more than once that my headaches, agitation, anxiety, depression, weight gain and low libido were ALL a result of stress. This has got to change. A doctor's education needs to trump an insurance company's underwriters.

So let's see, when my symptoms first started developing, I was in the military (USAF), stationed in (not-so) Grand Forks, North Dakota, working rotating shifts as an air traffic controller, raising a very active and energetic toddler with asthma and allergies, and playing the part of essentially a single mother with my husband across the state for work. As if that wasn't enough, I taught part time, was taking care of a one-year-old neurotic Dalmatian, working on finishing up my bachelor's degree, and on every other weekend, I would take my daughter on a three-hour road trip across the state to visit my husband. Would that cause anyone stress? Heck yes! It was easy for me to blame stress for all of my emotional and physical symptoms. To tell the truth, I was so exhausted most of the time that I didn't know what I was experiencing. Somewhere deep inside, I knew that I probably shouldn't be having all of the headaches I was having, but I just kept taking 800 mg of ibuprofen, every 4 hours. I was, after all, Super Mom, Wonder Wife and all around She Woman! Nothing could stop me...until years later that is!

Many other symptoms started to come up that I had also excused by blaming stress. Some I totally ignored, while others did indeed require medical attention. Unfortunately, even if you have all of the symptoms documented, putting the pieces of the jigsaw puzzle together for the proper diagnosis is difficult at best. My upbringing, growing up in a working middle class family from the Midwest also further delayed the diagnosis. You see, I was brought up to not complain about these little things. I didn't discuss many of what I thought were insignificant symptoms with my doctors because

I didn't think they were important enough, or even more to the point—I didn't think I was important enough. I was told more than once by my parents not to complain unless something was *really* bothering me, because doctors are busy treating really sick people and shouldn't be bothered by somebody healthy like me. Even worse, I may be given medicine that we couldn't afford. Feeling unworthy of a doctor's time was learned at a very early age and reinforced throughout my life.

This faulty thought process was further perpetuated by my military training, where being sick in any way is the same as being weak. The last thing you want to be thought of in any branch of the military is weak (OOH-RAH)! In addition to that, being an Air Traffic Controller means that you cannot legally take medications without being taken off of controlling status (not able to talk to or control aircraft) and forced into clerical duties. In the Air Force, I was seen by the flight surgeon (a doctor that only sees pilots and controllers). The basic prescription for most ailments the doctor saw was 800 mg of ibuprofen, given for pretty much any and everything you went there for. Anything stronger and you were taken off of flying/controlling status and had to follow-up with the doctor to be put back on controlling status. Too many trips to the flight surgeon looked bad, so I just learned to "suck it up," took the ibuprofen, and went on about my life. I was, after all, "a good airman" and "a good Midwestern girl" and had been trained my entire life to not complain about the "little things." A headache was a little thing after all, and I was under a lot of stress, so I saw no reason to give it another thought, right? After all these doctors were busy treating far more important people than me. People with *real* problems…

Then there is the female factor. As women, we are all told about the hormone changes that can easily explain away a lot of symptoms, like the ones that go along with having babies. Hormone changes can be the blame for: gaining weight, losing weight, swelling hands and feet, change in metabolism, depression, insomnia, irritability and I'm sure there are many, many other symptoms that match up with my Acro-symptom list. Now I had pregnancy and childbirth to blame a wide variety of symptoms on, in addition to the old favorite of being under stress. It was just plain ignorance for me, not knowing they were symptoms of something much more serious until I was diagnosed many years later. I really didn't even realize many of these irregularities were symptoms of another problem until long after diagnosis. Most of my physical changes were happening very slowly and weren't recognizable to me or those that were around me on a regular basis. Besides, my life was far too busy to recognize much of what was going on.

When my daughter was about eighteen months old, my husband and I decided she would be an only child. I was so over-extended and tired that I didn't feel like I could possibly care for another child. My husband and I agreed that I would get my tubes tied. During the surgery, my OB-GYN discovered I had a small fibroid the size of a grape that I should keep an eye on, but that they were very common. He said that these tumors could grow and cause irregular periods and heavy bleeding, and that if these things did happen, I should have my uterus checked for more tumors or changes in the size of the one that was present. This would become another tidbit I kept in the back of my mind to use later to justify symptoms or discount anything more serious or insidious taking place just below the surface. Some of my other acromegalic symptoms had popped up about this time and went unreported by me because they were either unpleasant or embarrassing, and really did not seem worthy of a doctor's time. Many of these symptoms included swelling and actual growing hands and feet, increased sweating with strong body odor, oily skin and mild adult acne, increased salivation, enlarging tongue, skin tags and some minor changes in facial appearance. I ignored these changes because I thought it was a "normal" occurrence because of aging, having a baby, or not losing the baby weight from pregnancy.

I got out of the military and changed jobs from Air Traffic Controller to college instructor for future Air Traffic Controllers. Soon after that, my husband and I purchased and moved into our first home. It would certainly take some time getting used to having my husband living in the same house again, and going to a civilian doctor for the first time in over eight years. I was starting to wonder if the stress machine would ever stop! While the machine may not stop, it does constantly change gears. My headaches were getting more severe and more frequent, to the point that they were pretty much constant if I didn't take the ibuprofen on schedule. I eventually changed to the cheaper over-the-counter approach after one of my doctors advised me that it would be the same if I just took four of the 200 mg generic or store brand ibuprofen. This now only took the edge off of the headache pain, but the yet undetected tumor was growing and the Acromegaly was becoming more active. I was still unaware that the small changes I was trying not to notice were the result of something worse that I didn't even know existed. The ibuprofen became less and less effective, and the headaches got worse.

Now that I was a teacher, I needed to have a professional portrait taken. When I got the proofs back and was told to choose one, it would be the first time I had seen a picture of myself in several years. As most parents know, after you have children, most of the photos taken are of their children, not the parents; and we were no different. When I saw the proofs, I was taken aback by what I saw! It seemed so surreal; I didn't look like Trena, if that makes sense. I didn't recognize my face as my own. My jaw seemed very different—more square, more pronounced; my brow area seemed puffy, and what happened to my nose? I always had a cute little nose, and now it was much longer and wider than I remembered with huge pores. When did that happen? Because of my pregnancy, it had been a few years since I really looked at myself in the mirror. I felt unattractive and blamed weight gain on the pregnancy. I asked my husband if the pictures looked like me and he said yes and that I was imagining things. He said I looked fine and just like I always did, and tried to reassure me that he thought I was still beautiful to him. Despite his loving reassurance, I still didn't think they looked like me, and I started noticing my deformities more in the mirror. I couldn't let go of the thought that I didn't look like me, or what I thought I should look like. Mentally, I would eventually let it go; and I gradually went back to not paying much attention to myself or my reflection. If you don't like it, avoid it, right? I did become more aware of my appearance in pictures. What was even harder was that I felt more and more distorted and unattractive with each photo, so I just avoided being in pictures as much as possible or made goofy faces to hide my real image. I made sure that I kept my time looking in the mirror to a minimum, so I could ignore what I didn't like seeing.

While the image issues were overrunning my mental well-being, my physical issues continued to grow worse. My headaches were getting more painful, and my body kept swelling. I was sweating more, and my appearance continued to change slowly over the next couple of years.

In 1997, I made another career move, this time to Minneapolis, MN. Moving meant new friends, and of course, new medical care with yet another doctor who didn't know my history, other than through the records I brought with me. When I went to my new doctor I told him of my headaches, and he asked me to describe the pain, a simple question that was a very pleasant change for me. I was more accustomed to a doctor who heard the word headache and wrote a prescription, told me to take Advil, or just straight dismissed it as stress. I explained my symptoms as the sensation of an ice-pick being stuck in the middle of the back of my head just below the skull and poking through the back of my right eye, along with a new symptom where my vision seemed to go grayish. Basically, it felt like I was viewing things through a tunnel with gray edges; mostly in the right eye. The doctor told me I had migraines, and I was put on a beta-blocker to regulate the blood flow through my brain. I continued on the ibuprofen regiment as well. All this helped ease the pain for quite a while, but the other problems were getting worse. I was still doing my best to ignore them, and I didn't fully discuss them with any medical professionals because I didn't want to be a bother or labeled as a troublesome patient.

Since having my tubes tied, about four years had passed. My periods gradually got worse and were to the point that I was having my period for twenty-one out of every twenty-eight-day-cycle. The first eight to ten of my periods were very heavy, and I had really bad cramps. I had really never had a "normal" period. Even in the beginning when I first started having periods, I had nine-day periods with very heavy days the first four days. Now, in addition, my sex drive was non-existent and had been gone for several years since childbirth. Who can feel sexy when they are having their period almost every day? I was so tired all the time and started being treated for depression. I tried a variety of different anti-depressant and anti-anxiety medications, but they only worsened the libido problems, and I was really worried that my husband would get sick of all of my difficulties and leave me. I felt like I was in a deep, dark hole and was getting sucked in further and further. I shared my thoughts and fears with my husband, and he suggested that I get more serious about taking care of myself now that our daughter was established in school. I was really afraid of what I might hear when I finally talked seriously to a doctor, so I did procrastinate a little bit longer, but I finally took my husband's advice and got myself checked out.

Before I really made the commitment to myself to get better care, I was relying on my family practice doctor to also provide my gynecological care. When I explained my situation, he referred me to a gynecologist for a more thorough examination from a specialist. During the first exam he told me I had several fibroid tumors, and at least one was the size of a grapefruit. We decided at that visit that I was going to have a hysterectomy that would leave one ovary. One ovary would keep me from needing Hormone Replacement Therapy (HRT). Even though HRT was the newest medical craze, I fought it. I followed my heart that kept telling me to keep one ovary and to avoid the HRT. It just seemed wrong to replace something chemically that the body could do naturally on its own.

On the day of the hysterectomy surgery, the doctor came out to let my husband know how everything went. He said he had to take one of my ovaries and that he had never seen so many tumors, *ever*. He explained to my husband then and to me later that I had them growing both inside and outside of my uterus. He said that one was attaching itself to my bladder and the others were putting pressure against my spine. He was sure that this is what was causing a lot of the back pain I had recently been suffering from. My husband asked how many tumors there were and the doctor's response was simply, "Too many to count." He commented that he had never seen anything like it. This left both me and my husband feeling shocked and feeling like it should have been taken care of before it got this bad.

Looking back now, I consider this a missed opportunity for early diagnosis. If the doctor said he hadn't seen anything like it, couldn't it have been a sign of something more serious? Numerous fibroid tumors are a symptom of Acromegaly. While I am not a doctor, I would love to think that this diagnosis would be seen as a possible reason to run lab tests for elevated Growth Hormone levels. Had I even the slightest clue that anything further was going on inside of me, I could have acted on it earlier and had a better chance at a cure, and I would hope that my doctor would give me the opportunity to make that choice for myself.

After the fibroid tumors were removed, I was hoping this was the magic bullet. That once I recovered from surgery, everything would fall back into place and I would feel normal again. Unfortunately, it was really just the beginning of my medical and emotional journey. The benefits of surgery were that I was done with having a period, and I could look forward to a normal sex life again. Moreover, I was thrilled that my lower back pain had virtually disappeared. Sadly, my libido never came back; but I will discuss this further a bit later.

Before I would officially be diagnosed with Acromegaly, I would have a few other smaller surgeries and procedures that, in hindsight, can be attributed to Acromegaly. They included diagnosis of bi-lateral carpal tunnel with surgical repair on the right wrist. This happened just after my hysterectomy. My carpal tunnel was really flaring up. I was originally diagnosed with this problem when my daughter was an infant, but I was told not to worry because many new mothers get this, and it would probably go away over time. It didn't. At this point, my daughter was about seven or eight and I was wearing splints on both hands at night and on the right hand through the day. The surgery gave me immediate relief from the tingling and numbness. Other procedures included laser hair removal on my abdomen and upper legs for a really weird hair growth pattern, a couple fatty tumors (lypomas) removed from my stomach and leg, and numerous skin-tags had to be frozen off.

Before, during and after all of my procedures, I have struggled with anxiety and/or depression, and I have felt like something was wrong; but I just couldn't pinpoint or explain it in a way that others could fully understand what I was saying. I didn't feel normal, even though I was living a normal life. I felt like a stranger in my own body. I could not understand how somebody in their mid-to late-thirties could be so tired and so completely worn out and apparently so done with sex. I tried several different medications for depression, but they all had side-effects that were frequently worse than the anxiety or depression, and most of the anti-depression medications worsened the low libido. There was one that I took that wasn't supposed to impact libido, but it turned me into such a raging monster that I feared physically hurting my daughter or being arrested for physically attacking someone. I remember worrying about this because I felt that I could lose control and fly into a rage, at any point and without reason. Where did all this anger come from? I stopped taking the depression medication and tried to manage on my own.

Emotionally exhausted and tired of battling depression, I was diagnosed with attention deficit disorder while getting my daughter screened for it, and we were both put on Ritalin. With this new prescription, the depression cleared up. I was much calmer and more focused than I can ever remember being in my entire life. I had energy when I took it in the morning and it stayed with me throughout the day, but the damn headaches were again returning and the low libido was still there. Again, at this point, I felt like this was the best it could ever get and it was better than I had felt in a long time. I would just deal with the headaches as long as I had energy. I was willing to compromise with my body. If I felt like a human being without the rage and emotional meltdown issues, the headaches were no big deal.

When I would go for my annual physicals, I complained about the headaches, and the doctor would tell me the theory of a boomerang headache. This is where you have a headache and you take medication to deal with it, but then the medication starts not to work and you get more headaches, so you take more pills, and so on. My doctor was pretty sure that was what was going on at this point with all of the years of my taking ibuprofen. I was asked to describe the pain again and used the ice pick analogy. This time I added a newer version of the old story because now I was dealing with deep jaw pain on the right side. I was told it was muscular at this point and was sent to physical therapy. Really?? I knew at that time, the pain was NOT muscular. I even tilted my head to the side as the doctor explained how the muscle in that area can cause the pain I described. What I should have told him right there was, "No way, dude! This is pain in my jawbone. It is deep in my jaw that is radiating from inside my head!!" But who was I to argue with my doctor? I knew before I even started that PT wouldn't work. This pain was inside my head and in my jaw joint and jaw bone below my teeth.

I followed my doctor's medical advice though and went to PT with no improvement. This felt like the biggest waste of my time for medical treatment. I stopped after three or four treatments even though I was scheduled for six weeks, twice a week. The therapist was sure my pain was all caused by a combination of my bad posture and weight gain. I knew that wasn't the cause, and I didn't feel any relief from the treatments. I decided I wouldn't mention my headaches to my doctor again, and I kept to that promise for a very long-long time because I feared another round of PT. In hindsight, I tend to wonder what kind of logic was I using? Instead of telling my doctor that the treatment wasn't working, I withheld the symptoms! What was I thinking?

More and more symptoms started appearing, reoccurring, or getting worse on a regular basis. I was sweating more and more with a really bad body odor; regardless of how often I showered or what antiperspirant I used. To rationalize this, I thought, "I know I have always had odor, and just need to use a stronger antiperspirant. It must be part of getting older or my hormones are changing again, right?" I thought it was probably due to my entering an early premenopausal state from the hysterectomy and having only one ovary. The sweating got so bad that I was embarrassed to go to the gym because I would sweat as much or more than the men. Women shouldn't sweat this much or smell this bad, I thought! I was worried about having armpit stains, and the more worried I got, the worse the stains got. I felt so gross and unfeminine that I became even more socially withdrawn. The only place I couldn't get away from this was at work, so I made sure I always wore a jacket or sweater. The problem with this was the smell that got embedded into the fabric. Again, I thought I smelled gross and I felt miserable, unfeminine and ugly.

If perspiring wasn't bad enough, I also started drooling—*a lot.* This was so disgusting and embarrassing to me. As a teacher, I was forced to deal with it in a public manner. I would joke and call the front row the spitting section and asked the students sitting there to reconsider their choice of seats. Little did most of them know, I was serious and I was scared to death that I would actually spit on them. One of the most humiliating things that happened was at a friend's house playing cards and talking, my saliva shot out like a cobra. It shot across the table hitting my partner's cards and hands. It was disgusting to say the least, but thank goodness I have friends with a great sense of humor, and we all laughed about it! But the fear of this happening in the classroom was causing me to lose sleep.

In addition to the increased saliva production, my tongue was also growing, making it difficult to speak clearly. I seemed to mumble a lot and appeared to develop some type of speech impediment, like a lisp. It seemed like my tongue got in the way of my ability to talk. I had a couple colleagues ask me if I was drunk on different occasions because of this speech problem. I tried to be very deliberate about what I was saying, but it all came out mumbling or mushy. I would describe it like what it sounds like when you're in the dentist's chair or you hold the end of your tongue still while you talk. This was humiliating as a teacher, and now I had to worry that co-workers or students could have thought I had a drinking problem.

Another embarrassment for me was my physical appearance. I started to gain weight slowly and without much change in my diet or exercise patterns. In a period of about three to five years, I went from weighing an average of 125 to 130 pounds to 165 to 170 pounds or from a size 6 to a size 12 or 14. The more weight I gained, the worse I felt about myself. Although, I was never a "girly-girl," as a woman, I still care about my appearance. While I was never vain or conceited before all of this started happening, in my own unique way, I felt pretty and confident. That confidence really took a beating as the physical changes took a toll on my self-esteem and confidence.

This disease has done a number on my self-image and my feeling of femininity. Looking at old pictures and comparing them with recent ones, there is a definite difference. The changes were not just from weight gain, there is something more to it. The structure of my face and entire body has changed to the point that when I looked in the mirror I don't see me or the me that I should be. It's hard to explain without sounding like I am in denial about the weight issue, but I know these changes weren't just a result of normal weight gain.

Because we moved to Minnesota soon after the onset of symptoms and before diagnosis, the people I saw every day didn't notice the changes. They didn't know what I used to look like and didn't understand when I tried to tell them about it. I used to have a longer, narrow face and now it was square shaped, much fuller, thicker in the bone around the jaw and eyebrows. My eyebrow area seemed puffier and while not painful appeared very swollen. My nose was wider and longer and my cheekbones were thicker and more pronounced. I was always described as small boned or small framed; but that was no longer true. My once thin fingers and dainty hands had grown puffy and appeared swollen all the time. Instead of having small or even normal girly hands, I had meaty farm girl hands, to the point that my rings had to be resized *twice*. My feet grew from a size 5½ or 6 to a size 7½ or 8 and are much wider than they once were. Most days I felt puffy and swollen like some sort of cartoon character; not very feminine at all. I don't fully know how to describe this, other than to again say I didn't feel or look like myself.

With the physical changes, I have also experienced some discomfort and real pains in my joints; even my bones hurt at times. My hands and feet still go numb or tingle to the point that it's very painful. My breasts are tender and have several cysts. At times I feel like a stranger in this body of mine. One of the most unwelcome, unflattering and unfeminine aspects of Acromegaly is skin tags. I have had over one hundred of them burnt/frozen off. I still have several skin tags around my bra area, under my arms and around my neck. When I say several I mean just that.

Up to this point I may have sounded pessimistic, angry or depressed. Often, I was all of those things at the same time. Mostly I felt like an old cliché—I was sick and tired of being sick and tired! I was probably pretty miserable to be around too. I remember hearing my husband say I am tired of coming home every day and seeing you so exhausted. This isn't the Trena I married. You have got to get this checked out. I want my old Trena back. I know she's there, let's get help and find her. So, one more time I listened to this wonderful voice of reason. I went to the doctor and told him the headaches were much worse and that I was in pain every day and I just wanted it to stop. I also told him I didn't want another prescription, I wanted answers. I explained that it felt like something was growing inside my head. I don't know what made me say that, but it got his attention, and he scheduled me for an MRI the next day.

Well, I had that MRI on a Thursday in the late afternoon and wasn't expecting to hear anything until the following week. Well I was wrong! We were playing cards with our neighbors at nine thirty on a Thursday night when my doctor called me at home and told me I had a mass on my pituitary called a *pituitary adenoma*. My head was reeling! Mass=Tumor. I also heard him say that this type was non-malignant and surgery would be necessary. In my shock, and trying to act calm in front of our friends, I tried to play it off and even joked around about it for the rest of the night. I heard nothing the doctor said after I heard tumor, and that's what I focused on. My doctor said I would be seeing a neurosurgeon soon so I joked that I wanted a good one and he said he had checked around and had one all lined up for me. The referral was for the top neurosurgeon in the Minneapolis area that dealt with pituitary surgeries. He was respected and very well known, so I was fine with this referral.

I was scheduled to go in the following week for blood tests and they confirmed the diagnosis of Acromegaly. The next day I began to do some internet research on the type of tumor I was diagnosed with and the surgical options that were available. This was in one word, OVERWHELMING!! There was not a great deal of information at the time. What was out there was specific and graphic. I learned terms like *Gamma Knife*, *staged radiation*, *trans-labial* and *transsphenoidal* and kept reading about this thing called Acromegaly. Well, I was convinced that this couldn't be what I had, but that is because I had glossed over the facts and concentrated my research on the surgery only. I was already in over my head and trying not to drown in the information or the emotions that were swirling within me. I knew I wanted to try the transsphenoidal approach because the whole thing just seemed to be a better deal: less invasive, less recovery time, and that was important to me—I thought.

Shortly after being diagnosed I was in the neurosurgeon's office being told that the best option for a cure was to have surgery. I already knew this. I was scared out of my mind but refused to let it show. Oh, who am I kidding, I was a nervous wreck and knew they could all see that. I stuttered and stammered through my questions and talked so fast I couldn't even hear what I said. They had to take my blood pressure 3 times and it was still high, which was new for me. Just the thought of seeing a "neurosurgeon" for a medical appointment had me freaked out. Being told that I "needed" surgery put my anxiety off the chart. I left that appointment in shock and don't remember a lot.

It was explained to me that my first surgery was going to trans-labial, going into the pituitary area under the upper lip, and over the top gum. I remember asking him about the trans-nasal procedure and he told me that I shouldn't risk it. That being a female, I wouldn't want to scar my face. This approach could and probably would leave a scar from ripping my skin from the nostril down to my lip. Well, with my being very naïve and with him being a Neurosurgeon, I felt stupid for even asking and was afraid to ask much more. I regret not pushing my agenda to this day. I live my life with few regrets, but this was one of them. I really wish I would have been more demanding or requested a second opinion. I now realize that this doctor was set in his ways and didn't want to learn this newer approach because he had always done it "his" way. I am also not very often intimidated by much, but the medical field and this whole brain tumor thing had me thrown for a loop and feeling I was at the mercy of the doctors' experience. When I got out to my car after this appointment I cried for the first time in years. I sobbed to the point where I couldn't breathe. These were big, ugly, nostril-flaring sobs! I was thinking "how," "why me," "why now," and "what am I going to do?" I cried until I couldn't cry anymore or passed out from not breathing. I can't remember. Thankfully nobody came near my car during that time. I was a mess! I strongly suggest having someone go with you to all of your neurosurgeon's office visits for emotional support and to catch things that you may miss because you will likely feel overwhelmed.

Never having any serious medical issues and only seeing the doctor once or twice a year, I was ignorant of the whole process. I really didn't know I had other options. I didn't want to chance making the doctor angry by asking for a second opinion. I was more scared than I had ever been in my life and felt lost, hopelessly lost. I tried not to show it or to let on that I was scared to my husband and to my daughter; I don't know to this day if I really pulled that off. I only allowed myself to cry again in the shower a couple of times a few days before this surgery.

I did do some more research on the internet about this whole thing to try to reassure myself that it was all going to be fine. During my visits to my doctor's office, we focused our discussions on the tumor itself, more than the diagnosis of Acromegaly. They didn't mention Acromegaly (or I didn't hear them mention it because I was FREAKING OUT) so I didn't concern myself with it. So, surgery is where my research was directed. It wasn't until much later that I realized that this surgery was only a starting point.

During my second appointment with neurosurgery, I was told what to expect in pretty thorough detail, but it still made no real sense to me. My husband went with me to this appointment just before surgery and we were again told what to expect. The following is what I remember the explanation to be:

"You will come to the hospital at 6 a.m., have an MRI/CT Scan, go through the pre-surgery check-in procedures. An IV will be started and you will meet your surgical team. Then we will take you into the room where your surgery will begin at 7:15. We estimate it to take 4-5 hours for the procedure itself. An incision will be made under your lip at the top of your gum line. This is where we will be placing tubes: one to allow us to see via a small camera and the other one will be used to remove the tumor. The tumor is basically the consistency of yogurt. So, we will mainly be using a vacuum-like suction device to remove most if not all of it taking 3-4 hours based on the size of the mass. We will be placing a metal "halo" on your head that will be screwed into your skin at the temples and in the back of your head. This will keep you from moving during the surgery. So, when you wake up you may have some blood in your hair in these areas. I don't want you to worry about the blood. After the surgery, we will have to clean and close you up, taking another hour.

Mr. Mathis, you will be given a pager and may stay in the waiting area, but may want to leave and come back later. We will let you know how it is going by calling you on your cell phone if you do decide to leave the waiting area.

We may need to harvest a small section of fatty tissue from your abdomen to close up the hole we make in the sinus, or if there is a spinal fluid leak. After the surgery, you will have a catheter in place for urination that will remain in place for most of your hospital stay. There will also be cotton packing in your nose that will stay in while you're in the hospital. Please try to remember not to touch this when you wake up. You will be numb and you could impact the healing process. When you wake up, try to remember to move as little as possible.

You will be in an intensive care unit for 24-48 hours after the surgery and nurses will check on you every 30 minutes. Try to sleep as much as you can in between these checks. It will be difficult but you will need to rest as much as possible and you will probably be in a great deal of pain. They will do their best to keep you comfortable and as pain free as possible. It will be important for you to communicate your pain level accurately each time they ask. During surgery, if there is a spinal fluid leak, we may need to use a lumbar drain. If we are required to use this you will be a bit more restricted and in more pain. You will not be allowed any visitors during your time in intensive care, except for immediate family.

You will be moved to another room about 48 hours after you get to the floor. Assuming everything goes well, and your pain stays manageable the nurse will still check on you, but less frequently. You will be encouraged to get up and walk around and to get as much rest as possible. You can expect to be in the hospital 7-9 days. Your cotton packing will be removed before you go home. The stitches under your lip will dissolve on their own. You will be numb from your nose down to your lip and part of your upper palette for 3-6 months, possibly longer. Some of this numbness may be permanent.

When you get home you will need to rest as much as possible. No straining and absolutely no lifting anything for several days and no exercising for at least 30 days. You won't want to do anything that will jar the pituitary. We will go over all of this again with your discharge paper work."

The explanation was pretty accurate, as well as scary, but I still had no real idea of what to expect. It was both better and worse than what I expected.

After they took me in for the surgery, my husband had a family friend come to meet him for breakfast, and he planned on doing some work since he was told it would be 4 or more hours until he would see me again. He was shocked when in the middle of breakfast the buzzer, like the kind they give you in a restaurant, went off signaling him to call. When he called they told him everything went better than expected. They got all of the tumor and that I would be in recovery in about 45 minutes and he could see me there. The surgery that was supposed to take 4-5 hours only took 45 minutes. Mark was thrilled but worried at the same time. As usual the neurosurgeon seemed confident that he was successful.

Something didn't seem right at the time, but we so wanted everything to be so successful that we didn't question it further and decided to trust him. To wake up without a headache or migraine at all for the first time in many, many years was awesome. That was all the proof I needed at the time. I was sure it was taken care of. Life was going to be normal again. YAY!!!!

When the doctor came to visit me I was again told that they got the entire tumor and the word "cure" was used. The lumbar drain wasn't necessary and they hadn't needed to harvest any fatty tissue to plug the hole that was made.

The worst part of this recovery was the noise in the hallways and nursing station. It didn't allow for any quality rest. The other weird thing was the removal of the nose tampon. Removing it didn't hurt, but it was the strangest feeling I have ever felt. It was gross! The relief of having it out was liberating!

The discharge and home recovery was just as mentioned and I returned to work about 4 weeks later and felt amazing! The recovery was much easier and better than I expected it to be. I felt pretty normal after leaving the hospital and was elated to not have any more headaches. I went back in for my follow-up visit a couple of weeks later and was told that everything looked normal and the word "cure" was used again. I was told that I would need to get a yearly MRI and visit with the Neurosurgeon annually after that for the rest of my life. Did I mention the headaches were gone … Halleluiah!!! No headaches!!

I didn't realize it then, but I am convinced that I should have been seen by an endocrinologist before and after the first surgery. As I mentioned earlier, Acromegaly was never really discussed by the surgeon, only the tumor and the surgery. I really had no idea that I had anything further to worry about. I went to my annual visit and was told everything still looked really good, and I was still unaware that I had the condition of Acromegaly. Then, about 6 months after that, 18 months after the surgery, the headaches came back with a vengeance. I went to see my family doctor and he scheduled an MRI and did the lab work. The tumor had returned, bigger than the original, and my GH and IGF-1 were higher than before. I returned to the original paper work and there and in my on-line records was that word that I had ignored and remained oblivious to –ACROMEGALY!!! Again, I went reeling into a downward spiral of emotions … This story was just starting.

This is where reality set in for me that I had this horrible thing called Acromegaly! This is also when I started to have a break down. I panicked and started a search on-line for Acromegaly content. There was too much but not enough! I didn't know what I was looking at most of the time. I began to realize the seriousness of this disease, the importance of GH/IGF-1 levels and why I was feeling so miserable for so many years and that there was little hope for an actual cure. I could feel myself spiraling. What was I going to do? How was I going to deal with this? How was I going to tell my husband and daughter it was back but worse? How was I going to get more time off of work? How could the doctor have been so sure he cured me and so wrong? How could he do that to me? How could this happen? Would my insurance cover this again?

I was referred back to the neurosurgery department, but asked not to be seen by the same doctor. I found out that the one I had previously seen had moved onward and upward to the Boston area. Good luck with that, Boston! There was some relief knowing that I wouldn't be going back to him. I was and am still very angry that the treatment I had already received didn't work. I also knew I couldn't just sit back and do nothing. So I went back and, as expected, I was scheduled for a second surgery.

This time the doctor was much younger, which initially concerned me. He showed me the MRIs from before the first surgery and the one just taken. He showed me the pituitary and the tumor, as well as the sinus wall where the hole would be made. He was very open to questions and was interested in what I was concerned about! Imagine that, he actually listened to me; the neurosurgeon listened to *me*! He was going through my nose instead of under my lips like I wanted for the first procedure. He also insisted that I go to an endocrinologist before the surgery because that's who would be taking over my long term care after the surgery was done. I was also scheduled with an ENT surgeon before the surgery since she would be assisting in the surgery.

He explained how having this procedure was different than the previous one and was genuinely pleased that I had done my own research. He even explained how the ENT surgeon would open up the sinus area and make way for him to get to the pituitary. He told me that this probably would not be a cure but was the best hope for one. It wasn't what I wanted to hear, but it was what I needed to hear. I was grateful for the honesty.

The endocrinologist I went to strongly advised removing the entire pituitary gland in order to stop the problem. I had never heard of this as a treatment anywhere in my research and I wasn't crazy about having to replace all the hormones. I certainly didn't want it to be removed if it weren't absolutely necessary. The endocrinologist was upset by this but he also understood my decision. So this surgery was done with the same basic explanation as the time before but through the nose. I was told that there was a greater chance of waking up with a lumbar drain, but had little understanding of what it meant as it was being explained.

This second surgery lasted about five hours. The ENT surgeon came out and kept my husband updated a few times during the procedure instead of him just getting a phone call. During this procedure, they used some fatty tissue from my abdomen to plug the sinus area. I had a 3-inch incision there just below and to the left of my belly button. There go all my bikini days (ha-ha-ha).

When I woke up after this surgery, I found that I had the feared lumbar drain and now realized quickly what he meant by "much more pain." I don't mean to scare anybody, but honestly, I have never experienced so much pain, EVER! The pain medication left me hallucinating and sweating profusely. I was tired but unable to sleep because my heart was racing from the amount of hydrocortisone I was taking just after the surgery. When I was able to sleep I had vivid, crazy dreams of being locked in a storage closet or on display in my bed in the hospital cafeteria. This was the most miserable I ever remember being. The nurses kept trying to get me to sit up in a chair for a few minutes but if I moved even the slightest bit I felt like my head was going to split in two. I honestly couldn't move for three days. I say these things not to scare anyone who is facing this, but to be honest with you. This pain was worse than the thirty-six hours of induced labor I endured giving birth! However, I will also say that I would gladly go through it again to have a chance at a cure.

After surgery, my GH and IGF-1 levels were taken and the results were shared with me after each lab. They didn't drop as much as they should have, so there was concern. The doctor knew and told us that he didn't get all of the tumor. He told us that there was residual tumor left and he couldn't get to it because the remainder was wrapping around the carotid artery and mixed with scar tissue from the previous surgery.

During my recovery, I developed diabetes insipidus. This is a miserable condition where your body doesn't absorb water and produces too much urine. This leaves you with an insatiable thirst and peeing every 3 minutes. This was the absolute worst case of cotton mouth I have ever had. No matter how much water I drank, I couldn't get to the bottom of the thirst. This was worrisome, but a wonderful prescription nasal spray alleviated these symptoms almost immediately. This condition resolved itself about 4 weeks later for me but in many cases is permanent. I was very happy that it cleared up.

During my hospital stay, I was monitored and cared for about the same about as well as I was during the first surgery and felt a bit more secure knowing the follow-up procedures. The lumbar drain was the worst part, and that was removed on the fifth or sixth day.

Having it removed made a world of difference. I felt better almost instantly and was able to shower and move about. My husband said he noticed a huge improvement as soon as he walked in that day. He said my eyes lit up and he said, "My Trena's back!" In the days before that you could see the worry in his face that I would never be myself again. I was scared myself, but just kept trying to rest and not worry. One minute at a time, I tried to just get through it.

The nasal packing was removed the same day and I was discharged the following day. The home recovery was easy, like the last time and I returned to work 3 weeks later. I went to my follow-up appointments, this time with my neurosurgeon, endocrinologist and ENT surgeon. I had a small infection at the incision sight and was given an antibiotic solution. My numbers were still not dropping after two months, so I was scheduled for a third surgery to have the entire pituitary gland removed this time just four months after the second surgery.

The third time went much the same way the second one did, but it took much, much longer. I was observed through an MRI several times during this operation. They started on me at about 7 am and didn't finish until about 6:00 p.m. I didn't get out of recovery until about 8:00 p.m. This is the only time I remember anything about the recovery room. The people who work there are wonderful.

I woke up again with a lumbar drain and a sizable 3- to four-inch incision on my outer right thigh from tissue removed to close the sinus cavity. This recovery was much better. I needed the lumbar drain again, but it didn't cause as much pain and I was able to get up and move around the second day. Instead of using nasal packing or a nose tampon, they inserted a rubber inflatable bladder to hold everything in place. In my opinion this was much better than the packing used in the previous two recoveries, which leaked and seeped. My GH/IGF-1 levels initially dropped but crept back up during the following days. On about the fourth day, I developed diabetes insipidus, again, as expected this time. We were informed that it would likely be permanent this time. The doctor also told us that there was still residual tumor left around the carotid artery that started bleeding when he tried to remove it. I thanked him for stopping and he appreciated my humor.

Before this procedure, I asked to have a different pain medication explaining the hallucinations and dreams. I am able to remember much more of what happened during this hospital stay. The other two are pretty foggy. I was more alert and aware of my surroundings and felt better. The pain was well managed and I felt pretty much myself after the second2nd day.

I was discharged with my nasal spray for diabetes insipidus, cortisone replacement and told that when I followed-up with endocrinology this time, I would probably begin taking thyroid hormone replacement. I could also opt to take female hormone replacement (estrogen) but decided not to and to just allow menopause to begin. Once again, the home recovery went well and I felt pretty normal, but a bit more tired this go round. My energy level continued to plunge as was expected because of a now non-functioning thyroid.

At my three-month follow-up appointment, I was placed on thyroid replacement hormone and my energy level increased. My levels GH/IGF-1 levels increased and I began taking self-administered injections three-times-a-day for thirty days to see if I could tolerate the medication. After the thirty days and tolerating it, I began the new drug therapy every four weeks and I am still taking them. Between the discharge date from the hospital and this appointment and much to everyone's amazement the diabetes insipidus had again resolved itself, which was great. During this visit to the endocrinologist, it was suggested that I take an over the counter supplement called DHEA in addition to the testosterone ointment to repair my libido. This has helped a little, but makes my hair and skin oily leading to acne outbreaks. To me the acne wasn't worth the limited success, so I reduced the dosage to half of a tablet. I still am getting very limited benefit but keep taking it hoping it will improve my libido someday.

My health care is still an intense balancing act and something that my medical team and I are still trying to perfect. My current drug therapy has known side-effects that I am dealing with that include: gastrointestinal upset and flatulence, gallbladder impairment, injection site pain, joint pain (knees and hips for me), sweating, and hypoglycemia (low blood sugar). For me, this normally happens after breakfast or before lunch, or with any physical exertion; to the point where I have to carry snacks with me at all times. As for the sweating, I am not sure if this is the medication or hot flashes from the onset of menopause, or both. I am having several (5-10) hot flashes a day in addition to just being hot most of the time. I am told that estrogen replacement would probably clear them up, but I am choosing not to take it because of the increased chance of breast cancer.

The things that have helped me emotionally and mentally are the on-line support groups I have found doing my research. I don't know where I'd be right now if I had not stumbled upon them. I have learned more from them than I have from the years of going to my doctors. I have formed many good friendships with others who have this and strongly suggest that anyone who has this or is close to someone that has it checks them out. My favorites are http://www.acromegalycommunity.com/ and http://www.dailystrength.org/c/Acromegaly/support-group. You can read others stories, ask advice, vent or lend support by sharing your story and experiences with other acromegalics around the world. They have made a huge difference in my emotional well-being and have been the source of a whole lot of good advice.

I still struggle with the toll these surgeries have had on my body and mind but refuse to surrender to it. After the surgery and recovery, I gained more weight and was heavier now than I ever was. I knew it was unhealthy and it was having an impact on my self-esteem as well. I knew that I could no longer blame it all on the surgeries or disease. When I was younger I never had trouble losing weight. I just cut down for a few days or a week and it was gone. It was much more difficult to lose this time. I have to wonder if it's age or Acromegaly. Either way I was determined to get healthy again. I joined a weight loss club, began working out again, joined a gym, and hired a personal trainer to help get me back into a healthy state of being. I feel better now than I have in over ten years and am approaching a normal weight and clothing size again. Losing weight, fitness and better health have helped improve my self-esteem, joint pain, mental attitude and energy levels. All the research out there seems to suggest that does so I will continue and am close to reaching my goals. Each day I wake up is a new beginning and I am glad to have the opportunity to experience it.

I have become a truly grateful person. I am grateful for what I have, what I've accomplished and what I've done and seen. Most of all I am grateful for the beautiful child that I was blessed with. She is amazing. Fertility is a real concern for many Acromegalics. You may be wondering if you can have children if you have been diagnosed with Acromegaly. For most people I have heard this is a possibility if the pituitary is still intact. I have no personal knowledge of this but it is a hot topic on the on-line support groups with lots of good information for those that are curious about this subject.

I am thankful that I have a wonderful, loving, understanding husband that is okay with me and the low sex drive aspect of our relationship. I am thankful that we did enjoy a normal sex life before having our daughter and this disease's onset. I mourn the loss of that part of our marriage. I was honestly relieved that it was largely because of the Acromegaly and it wasn't just something wrong me. It seemed to help me deal with the guilt to know that there was a medical condition that was causing the libido issues. There was and is a viable reason that I have no sex drive. I am still trying to get it back. It is important for me to reclaim this important part of my life. Adding the DHEA supplement has helped, but it still isn't what I would call normal. The DHEA can have some other side effects that aren't pleasant, like oily skin, and acne. I have found that taking half a tablet a day (one tablet is the recommended dosage) or every other day eases the side effects and still helps. I will continue to research this until I find something that works.

So far, my treatment has been three surgeries to remove the tumor and injections every four weeks to control my GH and IGF-1 levels. The injections continue taking my IGF-1 levels lower and this in turn manages the symptoms, but I am not cured. I have accepted it for now but have not given up hope. The way I have dealt with this chronic disease in my own life is with a lot of humor and as much knowledge as I can gain. I strongly believe that life is far too short to be miserable, unhappy and to not have fun. I find a way to laugh at everything and love to make people laugh. I feel strongly that every moment of my life is a miracle waiting to reveal itself. I am usually a pretty positive upbeat person with a strong sense of realism to balance the humor, but I still have dark times when I wish I had never heard of this disease and throw little pity-parties for myself. During these dark times, I am angry that I have this disease and have to take a painful shot or deal with the other medications, or struggle with low energy. To get out of these pity parties, I try to remember that it isn't as bad as some of the other things that are diagnosed every day. In those moments I am humbled and thankful and know that my life is worth living. I find that every time I have to walk the halls of the clinics at the University of Minnesota I see people in much more dire circumstances than my own, and I no longer feel sorry for myself. I also find meditation and daily affirmations helpful to keep myself from feeling sad.

The delayed diagnosis is a problem that I am trying to help solve. I have participated in and will continue to participate in patient panel groups for the drug manufacturers. I will aid in any book project or documentary that will bring light on this mystery and do what I can to help my fellow Acromegalics get the treatment they need. These patient panels and on-line support groups have broadened my circle of friends and have helped me out of some dark times. I may also volunteer for clinical trials to help find better treatments for all of us. So far that opportunity has not presented itself. I am always looking for ways to serve and better myself and help others. My advice to anyone facing this is to find a way to tap into some type of spiritual practice. Some of you may find strength or comfort in religious practice and a house of worship, or by meditation, prayer or some other avenue. This to me is the most essential part of my recovery. I have found books by Dr. Wayne Dyer and Eckhart Tolle to be most helpful in being happy during challenging times. I personally have found a great comfort in the many translations of the *Tao Te Ching* by Lao Tzu. Any spiritual practice may bring you comfort and understanding when you need it the most. Quiet time for praying/meditating was essential to repairing my emotional balance.

In closing my chapter I would like to leave you with something that I have posted in many places—in my bathroom, in my office, on my computer—that helps me during times of stress or grief. I found this on one of the on-line support groups. It has become my motto and I hope it helps you:

> Believe in your heart that something wonderful is about to happen.
>
> Love your life.
>
> Believe in your own power, and in your own potential, and your own innate goodness.
>
> Wake every morning with the awe of just being alive.
>
> Discover each day the magnificent, awesome beauty in the world.
>
> Explore and embrace life in yourself and in everyone you see each day.
>
> Reach within to find your own specialness.
>
> Amaze yourself and rouse those around you to the potential of each new day.
>
> Don't be afraid to admit you're less than perfect; this is the essence of our humanity.
>
> Let those who love you help you; Trust enough to be able to take.
>
> Look with hope to the horizon of today, for today is all we truly have.
>
> Live this day well.
>
> Let a little sun out as well as in.
>
> Create your own rainbows.
>
> Be open to all your possibilities, and all miracles.
>
> Always believe in miracles.
>
> (Author unknown)

Trena Mathis, M. Ed., is an Air Traffic Control Instructor at Minneapolis Community and Technical College (MCTC) in Eden Prairie, MN. She earned her master of education from the University of Minnesota. She has been teaching air traffic control (ATC) at MCTC for over 13 years. Before MCTC, she also taught ATC at the University of North Dakota and served in the United States Air Force for over 8 years as an air traffic controller at the Berlin Air Route Traffic Control Center, Tempelhof Airport, Berlin, Germany and Grand Forks AFB, ND as a tower and approach controller. This is her first experience with writing.

Talking with Your Children
Collaboration of Acromegaly Community Members

Maria King
St. Louis, MO

I did not have the energy to really play with my children all the time before and of course even after my diagnosis with Acromegaly. As most of us know and accept, it is a chronic condition that we deal with. It can be managed, but it can still affect our day-to-day activities; and the well-being of my children was becoming more and more of a concern to me. My children are now 10, 8 and 4. I would like to share my FOCUS that allowed me to use my time wisely. My diagnosis, looking back was a true gift. It made me realize even more how precious each second is that God gives to me. Taking care of our children has always been my focus but I did have to learn that in order to take care of them, I needed to first take care of myself and my health: mind, body and spirit. I do this by remembering to FOCUS. I also will share with you what each of these letters in the word means to me and how it has helped me in taking care of my children over the past six years since my diagnosis.

First I Know You Must Put the Large Rocks into Your Jar.

I remembered the story about putting large rocks into your jar first and then filling it with sand. I remembered that if I put the sand in first, my rocks might not fit. I realized to raise my children and still take care of myself I needed to follow this plan. I made a list of my rocks. These rocks were things like cooking healthy family meals, getting daily exercise, engaging with my children in active play, going to church together, and needing to add in date nights with my husband.

My sand was house cleaning, excess shopping, and all the other little stuff that was really not all that important. My sand was also trying to write. My son has always told me I should write my story so that I did not forget it. The saying that it only takes a spark to get a fire going is one that I told him, and he made me remember; my child helped me to put my pen to paper.

Offer Help to Others.

As a mother I learned after my diagnosis that I needed to teach my children the importance of helping others. I wanted to teach them by example just how important it was to volunteer. I feel that this gives each and every one of us a sense of purpose.

I started to volunteer as an ice skating instructor. I had skated as a child and teen; but as an adult, I had to buy two pairs of skates in four years because my feet kept growing, so eventually I just remained off the ice. When I got back on the ice and my children saw me doing something I loved, and they saw me smile, the message was clear to them. I cannot explain just how pivotal this was in my recovery process. Return to something you love to do. Replace all your memories that are not so good with new, happy ones. Slowly but surely in time those not so happy ones will fade. I had a new normal after my diagnosis but one I was happy to accept. I am now an ice skating pro and am teaching ice skating lessons four months out of the year. I fit a new, important rock in my jar, volunteering to help others. It landed me a wonderful job that has continued to bring me joy each time I step onto the rink.

Can-do Attitude.

I have tried to pass this—a can-do attitude—onto my children with the following tale:

You are what you believe about your self – author unknown

One day a naturalist who was passing by inquired of the owner why it was that an eagle, the monarch of all birds, should be confined to live in the barnyard with the chickens.

"Since I have given it chicken feed and trained it to be a chicken, it has never learned to fly," replied the owner. "It behaves as chickens behave, so it is no longer an eagle."

"Still," insisted the naturalist, "it has the heart of an eagle and can surely be taught to fly."

After talking it over the two men agreed to find out whether this was possible. Gently the naturalist took the eagle in his arms and said, "You belong to the sky and not to the earth. Stretch forth your wings and fly." The eagle however was confused. She did not know who she was. (This was me before Acromegaly diagnosis.) Seeing the chickens eating their food, she jumped down to be with them again (back to being exhausted and depressed and symptomatic). Undismayed, the naturalist took the eagle on the following day up on the roof of the house and urged her again, saying, "You are an eagle. Stretch forth your wings and fly." But the eagle was afraid of the unknown and jumped down once more for the chicken food.

On the third day the naturalist rose and took the eagle out of the barnyard to a high mountain. There he held the monarch of birds high above him (this is what my great doctors did to me … they said … You have to live your live again!!!!!) and encouraged her again saying, "You are an eagle. You belong to the sky as well as the earth. Stretch forth your wings now and fly."

Then the earth began to tremble; slowly she stretched her wings (slow and steady I began to trust doctors again after my diagnosis, and slowly I began to live my life again). At last with a triumphant cry she soared into the heavens. (For me seven years after my diagnosis I am living a quality of life I would have never known without encouraging friends and brilliant doctors who cared for me.)

It may still be that the eagle still remembers the chickens with nostalgia; it may even be that she occasionally revisits the barnyard. But she has never returned to live the life of a chicken (my life before my diagnosis).

Just like an eagle, if you have learned to think of yourself as something you aren't, you can re-decide in favor of what you really are. In truth, you really are an eagle with the potential to soar, to be FREE (of Acromegaly) and experience your real essence. But alas, you find yourself in the chicken yard feeling safe, but with no sense of purpose or direction. (Know if you are ever still sitting in the chicken yard that there are many of us with Acromegaly that are here for you … we have been there too.)

Understand Yourself.

I have tried to teach my children that they will be at their best when they understand themselves. What are their strengths? What are the areas where they are not so strong? I have had to look at myself and ask myself these same questions. Once you recognize them you can balance them as well. This was key for me as a parent with Acromegaly. I had to really look at how my strengths had changed after my diagnosis. I used to be the best listener. I now became one who only asked questions. I used to trust everyone. I soon trusted no one. All of these changes came for me as a parent, and I had to really look and think, Do I want to pass this onto my children or do I want to learn to listen and to trust again? A few years after my diagnosis I did find balance and that balance too has helped me in every aspect of my life.

Stay on Track.

In child rearing I have found it important to try to stay on track. However, you need to be on the right one and you need to keep moving. I was told once that if something is not dead, it has to be alive. If something is alive it is growing. I keep this in mind when trying to stay on track. Am I growing in the direction I want to? How am I growing? I ask the same questions now in every aspect of my children's lives. Again, going back to wasted time.

There are a Few Areas I learned to Stay on Track and to Never Quit.

Medical: Search until you find the right answer. I heard this lesson loud and clear after my diagnosis. This is one lesson I will always remember and will remind my children daily to always keep looking for answers. Remember that even though you may have one answer and that it might be correct, there could always be another answer that could come along that could be even better in some ways.

School : Knowledge is power and slow and steady win the race.

Exercise: The song that sums it up for me and my kids is "You've Got to Move It, Move It." I have also taught my children about FOCUS through exercise. For one hands-on activity that I like to play with them, I toss ten tennis balls at them at once and see how many they catch, then five, then one. Usually they only catch one each time and sometimes they miss all except the last one thrown singly. I ask, Why did this happen? They figure it out.

Perspective.

I will end with a story my Father always tells me that makes me remember what the neurosurgeon told me when I was diagnosed. I was told that of all the brain tumors I could have, mine was the best one to have. Kind of cold comfort; and I did not understand that at that moment, but now I get it. Perspective is so very important.

So the story is about two children. One was given a room full of new toys. The other child was given a room full of cow manure. At the end of the day, the child in the room full of toys was bored. The child in the room with the manure was still happy and looking around saying that with all this manure, there had to be a horse in there somewhere.

I love to share these stories with my children.

I always remind my children that with all things in their lives that might be difficult, to enjoy rainbows, you have to wait until after the rain. Looking for the rainbows is such a joy with all three of our beautiful children!

As a parent, one of the key lessons I learned from my *medical adventures* is that saying "I'm sorry" and saying "I forgive you" are important lessons for my children to learn. I realized that even as a mama of three and a mama with her master's degree in education, not knowing how to forgive almost killed me and would have done so quicker than my pituitary tumor.

I have also learned that although doctors are trained in all the information about the body and how to heal us physically, not all of them have the bedside manner that allows them to say I am sorry if they do guide you in the wrong direction or spin you in circles before you receive a correct diagnosis. My uncle is a doctor who had told me very politely after my surgery that the dance with doctors is complicated. Sometimes you need to lead and sometimes you need to follow. The tricky part is knowing when to do both. I have found and am still figuring out how to trust first and second guess second. I am finally learning to forgive the doctors in the past who could not acknowledge that they could have listened to me more and possibly found my proper diagnosis if they would have not excused my symptoms as the stress of being a new mother who was overwhelmed.

I hope I can pass onto my children a lesson that I have learned on walking the fine line without falling off. The dance of leading and following your doctor. Knowing when to lead, and knowing when to follow. Knowing when to listen and knowing when to question. Even the smartest person does not know everything they say, but the person who knows which question to ask and who to ask is most wise. A lesson to pass on…

The following is a blog excerpt printed with permission from Alecia E. from http://blessed-beyondmeasure.blogspot.com.

Day Before Surgery

"I'll see you in the morning, Mommy..." my three-year-old daughter said to me as I prepared to leave for Los Angeles the day before my surgery. It was those words that inspired me to write this next entry.

Saying goodbye to my husband and the kids before the surgery was really difficult. Although Dr. Kelly had only had one person out of 500 surgeries that had died as a result of the surgery, there was a chance that something could go awry...I knew I needed to prepare for the worse. My husband and I decided to leave our kids with my in-laws while we went to stay overnight near the hospital. When it was time to leave I sat down with each of my kids individually and had a talk with them just in case it was the last time we saw each other. I wanted to assure them that "if God decided to take Mommy to heaven" or if I didn't come home right away that they needed to try to accept it. My older two kids understood as best as I think they could have, but when it came time to talking with my youngest daughter she replied she'd "see me in the morning." Nothing I said could help her understand that in the morning I would not be here... and I wasn't sure when or if I'd be back.

Here is an excerpt from a letter I left for my husband in case he came back to Texas without me:

"I feel kind of silly writing a letter in case I don't make it out of surgery, but I would hate to go and be with the Lord and not have any final words to say. Since on this side of the operation it is difficult to know what the outcome will be, I hope this will be a letter we can laugh about and toss in the trash when we get back from California. But if that doesn't happen . . . I wanted to tell you goodbye one more time.

All of this tumor stuff has caused me [to] reflect seriously about my past and the changes in my life that have occurred since you and I met and married. This month is the anniversary as to when I became a Christian, August 2, 1992. I would have never thought I'd be confronted with death at such a young age. I thank God he changed my life when he did. God has given me full and complete joy through our marriage, your love, and in raising the children. These truly have been the happiest days of my life . . .

It's an awkward feeling to know that I might leave this life at such a busy time. If it were up to me, I'd stick around. I've got some unfinished work to do! But God's plans are not always what we expect and I hope, in time, you will accept this...I am praying for you now, that God would help you through this time should it turn out to have a tragic ending. Remember, there are no goodbye's in Christ."

Michelle French
Ridgefield, WA

When I was first diagnosed with the tumor, all I knew was that I had a pituitary tumor and was going to be going through several tests to find out more about it. I found out December 2008; at the time my children were 2 ½ years old and 7 years old. After several tests, it was found that it was secreting growth hormone.

Initially I told them both that there was something in mommy's head that wasn't supposed to be there and that the doctors were just going to keep taking pictures of my head and checking my blood.

By the time the doctors and I decided surgery was necessary, nearly a year and a half had gone by, putting my youngest at just 4 years old, the oldest at 8 ½.

We still kept it simple with the youngest, telling her that in order for mommy to stay healthy I had to have the doctors take the "thing in my head" out and that I would be in the hospital for a few days. We made sure she understood that as soon as the doctors said I could home, I would, and that she would be able to stay with her aunt and grandma while I was in the hospital.

We gave more details to the oldest. He was scared of me having the operation so we explained to him what could happen to me if I didn't have the surgery— that I might not live as long, that my organs could be growing, and that I could have other health issues. He also asked if it was cancer. We told him that these tumors usually are not cancerous. We also told him that once it was removed, I might not have headaches anymore. He wanted to know details of how they got it out, so we explained to him how they can go through the nose. I told him that the neurosurgeon had done this same operation for several years, and I had my son come with me to meet the ear, nose, throat surgeon that would also be helping with the operation. I showed him the MRI pictures and identified parts. He wanted to know if he would be able to see me after the surgery or be able to talk to me or if I could tell him good-night each night I was away. We also gave him a choice of whether or not he wanted to be at school the day of my surgery. I always asked him if he had questions that either I or the doctor could answer for him.

I am now 2 ½ weeks post-surgery and recovering well. I think being honest, yet simple and age appropriate when explaining the details to my children worked well.

Kathy Kurtz, MSW
Kathy is a social worker with many years of experience working with individuals and families facing medical and emotional issues. We thank her for her willingness to contribute her experiences and knowledge to our effort.

As the above stories reflect, dealing with medical issues is difficult enough on its own, and becomes even more complicated when thinking about how to tell one's children what is happening. Whether it is illness, divorce, or any serious issue, children essentially want to know three things—"Is it my fault?", "Can I catch it?", and "Who will take care of me?" If a parent is ill, children will need to be reassured that nothing they did or said caused the illness, that it is not contagious (they can still hug and kiss their parent as usual), and that when needed, they will be cared for by other adults who love them and will keep to their normal routines as much as possible.

There's often an instinct as a parent to protect one's children and to want to shield them from difficult news or situations. However, children are perceptive and notice when there are more phone calls, more doctor appointments, more hushed conversations. By including children and telling them basic information that is age appropriate, much anxiety will be avoided. Encouraging children to ask questions and even to visit the doctor's office are great ways to help children truly know what is happening, rather than leaving it up to their imagination.

In addition, it is important to allow children the opportunity to express their feelings about what is happening without being criticized. Perhaps they are angry that a parent missed one of their soccer games or sad that a parent is too tired to play with them. Cries of "It's not fair!" may be heard, and the child simply wants to hear, "You're right. It's not fair." Providing activities such as drawing or writing in a journal may also be helpful, as will taking a team approach: "We will all deal with this together as a family, and we will include you and let you know what is happening as we know it."

Remember that you are the one who knows your children best – you will be able to tell if they are experiencing changes in sleep, appetite, behavior etc. Most of the time, children will hear news that might make adults sad or scared, but their response is "okay, can I go play now?" As long as they know they can talk to someone, ask questions, and be included, they will take much more in stride than we sometimes give them credit for. If they do experience a more serious reaction or response, there are professionals with whom they, or the whole family, can speak. Children are resilient, and often look to their loved ones for guidance in how to respond to a situation – if the adult is matter-of-fact and coping well, the child will learn from this behavior. That being said, it is perfectly fine for a child to see an adult cry or express frustration, and to know that those feelings are part of the overall experience. We can't always protect children from difficult situations, but we can help them learn how to cope and respond.

Managing Disease Symptoms

Collaboration of Acromegaly Community Members

Editor's Note: This chapter is a very different and very special chapter. It has been written by a number of patients dealing with the effects of Acromegaly, who wanted to share their stories with you. They are discussing their navigation of the effects of Acromegaly. I tried to do as little as possible to their stories to make sure that it was their message that was communicated. Please appreciate these people for how great they are to share their lives with all of us. I hope you learn as much from them as I have.

Maria King
St. Louis, MO

June 9, 2003, after attending a sorority pledge class reunion, my pledge sister who is a pediatrician, called me and said that I looked different. She had not seen me in almost seven years. I immediately started to cry because I knew something was wrong. She said that my face, hands and feet all looked different and my voice had changed; it had gotten deeper. I immediately started to tell her that my doctor had put me on diacritics intermittently for the past three years to try to treat the swelling of my hands and feet. Then we talked about my shoe size, which had gone from an 8 1/2 to an 11, and my ring size increasing. We talked about my headaches, dizzy spells, sweating, drips of milk coming out of one breast, and major fatigue; all of which I had been having for years. She said, "I think you have Acromegaly." She said that I needed to get an MRI to be sure, so we got off the phone, and I immediately called my family doctor. I did have an MRI that same day and my friend was correct. I had a pituitary macroadenoma.

Then, my friend, although she lives out of state, directed me to one of the best hospitals in the world for neurosurgery. The neurosurgeon I saw listened to me and explained to me what was happening. I was in a state of shock but was listening to every word as he gave me his recommendations: transsphenoidal surgery and then possibly Gamma Knife and a medication called Sandostatin. It was such a relief to be diagnosed and know what was wrong with my body. I had been searching for answers for so many years that I was ready to aggressively treat this tumor which had been destroying my life.

I was scheduled for transsphenoidal surgery on June 26th, 2003. Surgery went very well, but the follow up MRI still showed residual tumor. My neurosurgeon suggested that I try medication and then have Gamma Knife radiation.

I was scheduled for Gamma Knife but then postponed it for a couple of months, rescheduled and almost postponed it again. In that time I did research on the Gamma Knife and started the medication Sandostatin which lowered my growth hormone Levels. I knew that although I could stay on medication for the rest of my life, I was only 30 years old and preferred to continue with aggressive treatment, so I called once again to get back on the schedule. I was still very anxious because I did not like the idea of being awake during this procedure. I am thankful that it was not at all as bad as it looked.

On the day of my treatment, to reduce my anxiety, my doctors and nurses gave me lots of reassurance and a little bit of medication. The frame placement was not as painful as I expected and once the frame was on, I felt no pain at all. It was like wearing a hat you cannot take off. It looks so painful, even to look at a picture today; but I was truly in no pain at that time at all.

As far as the MRI that I had after the placement of the head frame, it was no big deal either. I have become claustrophobic since I was introduced to the MRI machine, but once again, it was all ok. Charlotte, my Gamma Knife nurse, was right by my side during the entire MRI, and I could always talk to the doctors and nurses during the entire Gamma Knife procedure. Just knowing someone was always there made me comfortable, and time went fast. When the procedure was complete, the doctors removed the head frame and I think I was really light headed from the release of the pressure. All my doctors and nurses were still right by my side, and within minutes I was with my husband in amazement that the procedure was over. After just a short time I was then released and went to eat lunch in the hospital. My friends and family laughed that it took me an hour to realize I could move my head around even after the head frame was off. I was in no pain at all and felt great!

I cannot say enough about the nurses and doctors at the Gamma Knife. This procedure is a key part of treating the tumor that could have taken my life if it was not found and aggressively treated. I am looking forward to the day I see my MRI results with no tumor in sight. I am so thankful for the quality of life that has been given back to me. My mind, body and spirit have been healed. I am truly blessed to have such a wonderful team of medical professionals. Thank You!

Finally a Diagnosis
Rochelle Buckley

I have been struggling with pain, especially in my joints, for some years now; my vision, although I wear glasses is often blurred. My skin is incredibly oily and although I feel like I have tried every diet known to mankind, I continue to pile on weight. I have been complaining for several years that my feet are growing, but I thought it was just because I have been putting on so much weight. My shoes needed to be replaced every season for the last three years; my shoe size has gone from an 8 to a 14. My hands have also grown, again, I thought that it was just the weight gain. Even my face has changed, again I was thinking it was weight gain, but my cute little nose has become quite fat.

In January this year (2009), I drove to Queensland with my 13-year-old daughter for a holiday. It was fabulous but I found that each day I was becoming increasingly tired, exhausted and sore all over. Yet again I was putting it all down to the weight gain. The trip back home became quite difficult as I was enduring extreme joint pain and numbness down my left side: my left arm was all pins and needles and my left leg and my toes were just numb to the point that I couldn't feel them at all.

I made an appointment with my general practitioner, who I hadn't seen for about 8 months, and he sent me off for an enormous set of blood tests, telling me he thought I had Ross River Fever but wanted to check everything else out so he could be on the safe side. A few days later, I received a phone call from him, on a Saturday, from his home asking if I could see him at his office first thing Monday morning. **"Alarm Bells."** Of course I worried all weekend.

When I got to his office he sat me down and asked to look at my hands, then my tongue and then he looked over my face. He asked me if I had heard of Acromegaly and I responded with a no. He continued to give me a brief explanation of what it was and said he wanted to send me off for more blood tests. These tests had to be done in a government department as they did more extensive screening than the private pathologists I had been to. These tests came back positive so I had to be admitted to hospital for blood to be taken every 30 minutes for 4 1/4 hours, a total of 9 lots of bloods taken. Well it was quite traumatic. Don't get me wrong, I am not afraid of needles; I can cope with the poking and prodding and even the sight of the blood but they just kept sticking me. I asked for a butterfly canula so they wouldn't have to find a vein each time they needed to draw blood but they wouldn't do it. (I think they were teaching that day!) Anyway, we were about 1/2 way through the test and my bladder was so full of water after drinking 2 1/2 liters while I was there and my veins collapsed. I was stuck 29 times that day before being sent home as they were finished. If I had known it would be that hard and my body would have reacted the way it did, I would have had someone drive me home.

After all of these tests came back positive, I was sent off for an MRI, which of course was not so straightforward, as I am so obesely overweight that I wouldn't fit in any regular MRI machine. Thankfully a brand new MRI, a bigger one, was being installed at a nearby hospital, so I went there and actually fit inside. The MRI showed a pituitary macroadenoma - a tumor which sits under the brain and behind the eyes. It grows on the pituitary gland and causes the body to produce too much human growth hormone, or HGH.

In some ways it is such a relief to get a diagnosis. It is a relief to know there is a reason that I can't get this weight off, and why I am in so much pain all the time. So many people have told me over the last few years that I should be disgusted in myself, why can't I just lose weight; don't think about it just do it. Stop complaining about being in pain, just deal with it, buy some timber, build a bridge, and get over it. Now I understand it is not like that, I am not like everyone else, the pain is not like what other people I know would experience.

Before long I would have to leave work because it got to be too much; in fact I left work before I knew what was wrong. I resigned in December 2008 because I couldn't handle the pain, the tiredness, the exhaustion. I only worked Thursdays and Fridays and it was taking me until Monday to recover from two days work.

I have experienced facial swelling of my nose, my eye lids and my lower lip. My face in general is just all fat and puffy. I have skin tags on my chest and breasts and under my arms, only small ones but they are still there. I have terrible pain in my joints; my feet and ankles are probably the worst. I guess that is because they are supporting so much weight. Some mornings I get out of bed and when I stand up I immediately crash to the floor because the pain in my ankles and feet feels like they have been shattered.

I am beginning to experience difficulty speaking because my tongue feels very thick and fat I guess is the best way to describe it, and it really seems to cause me difficulty pronouncing certain words. I feel like I get all tongue tied and sometimes I just can't spit out the words, I just can't pronounce them and it is a bit like I am stuttering. It's a bit like my tongue is in the way, it is just too big.

I am noticing my memory is deteriorating too; some days I can't remember what I did 5 minutes before; sometimes I can't remember much at all. I forget whole conversations like they never happened. I thought everyone around me was going mad, but it is me. I honestly don't know if the memory loss is due to the tumor or just the whole stress thing. There is so much going on in my life right now that maybe my brain is just too full.

Sure, finding out you have Acro is enough but before diagnosis we already had a number of issues including problems with the children and their father, multiple deaths in the family, and cancers in other family members. It's just life and sometimes it just comes at you all at once and gets a little overwhelming. Maybe this is the contributing factor to my memory loss. I get **EXTREMELY** tired, irritable, and cranky. As much as I try to be happy, positive and energetic, it feels like it just won't happen.

I am beginning to battle depression and finally started anti-depressants. It is all getting a bit too heavy to manage. Of course I have good days, really good days with little or no pain, I move around with ease, I can remember things, I can function with a feeling of general normalcy—the next day it all comes crashing down where I am in complete agony, needing pain relief and sometimes unable to even walk. My memory disappears, I can't talk properly; it is so very frustrating.

My eyesight is getting increasingly blurry and I am constantly cleaning my glasses thinking they are dirty; since my skin is so incredibly oily, it gets all over my glasses. I had an eye exam recently, expecting to have to get a new prescription, thinking I would be able to see clearly again, but the optometrist informed me that my eyes have not changed in the last two years. I was devastated and demanded to know why I couldn't see clearly. He explained to me he could see the tumor pushing on the front of the optic nerve, was causing the blurriness. He told me there was good news in here—once the tumor is removed, I should regain full eyesight.

I would go to sleep and sleep for 12 to 14 hours and wake up exhausted. Some nights I would wake up gasping for air; it was quite frightening. I found out I had sleep apnea; this was the first of my symptoms to be diagnosed. I sleep now with the help of a CPAP machine but some days I still wake up exhausted.

My perspiration has gotten terrible. It used to be that I would use deodorant; it would last until my next shower—not now. I perspire like crazy and have to reapply deodorant several times a day. This makes me feel horrible, dirty, even like I have no respect in myself, so some days I just stay inside and don't want the world to see me.

I think the worst part is that I just don't feel like myself anymore. I can't find the right words to tell anyone just how I feel. I get incredibly frustrated; along with the pain and exhaustion I feel, I fear that my family and friends must get incredibly frustrated with me as well. They invite me out to functions or even just out for coffee and I always tell them yes, I would love to come, but sometimes I wake up that morning and just can't get out of bed.

It is only now with the diagnoses of Acromegaly that these ailments are beginning to make sense. Although my endocrinologist tells me I should not be experiencing all this pain, from reading of other experiences, it seems to be quite normal.

Kit DiMambro
Female, 58 years old
Diagnosed 5/2008, they say I probably had it 5–7 years

When asked to consider writing about my feelings, emotions and physical issues regarding my Acromegaly disorder, I thought I might have something to share, but I didn't want to be part of a book. I am a very private person, who is still to this day very uncomfortable and embarrassed by my diagnosis.

I told only my family and 2 friends. To this day, I rarely discuss it with anyone.

I am a 58-year-old female, diagnosed at age 56 in May of 2008. I was told I probably had it between 5–7 years, maybe even 10 years. Prior to ever hearing the word Acromegaly or knowing what it meant, I had some ironic conversations with my sisters. Just little comments regarding things about myself I wasn't happy with. It was what I was noticing and feeling "ugly" about. I made comments like, *I really hate my nose, has it always been this huge?* I would say that *my voice sounds like a guy's, people mistake me for my husband on the phone. Have I always sounded like a man?*

When I would wake up, I scared myself. I thought I looked so much like a "monster." And I wasn't kidding. I wondered why so many things hadn't bothered me before now. Was this a midlife crisis? When I looked at current photos of myself, I couldn't believe it was me. This disorder has turned my self-image into Frankenstein. To confirm my feelings, just check out the "famous people" with Acromegaly on the internet. Then you know what I mean. *Had I changed this much? Why?*

There were additional "masculine" attributes. My husband claimed I snored louder and harder than a trucker, all night long, and would seem to stop breathing for seconds at a time. He insisted I see a doctor. I brushed it off like everything else. I saw myself in the sunlight and saw more facial hair (thank god it was blonde) than a man. My feet were as big as a man's now, growing from a size 8 to a 10 1/2 or 11; and my hands not only were large, chubby and wrinkled, some of my knuckles were large and disfigured.

My skin had became very porous and course, and I was fighting pimples and blackheads. At one point I had so many little bumps on my neck (turned out to be skin tags) I pinched and squeezed them off myself. My face had creases instead of wrinkles, and puffiness under my eyes. What the heck is this all about?

Because of my embarrassment, I kept a lot of health issues to myself. I didn't share them with <u>anyone</u>. My excessive sweating had no odor, thank God, but my underarms were always wet. Well, I assumed stress was involved.

Dawn Canright

...Notsureexactlywheretobegin...cameacrossAcromegalyCommunity.com after an all night, frantically rigorous exploration on this strange thing called Acromegaly...

...I have known for several years now that something was amiss in my body...wasn't sure if it was due to metabolic changes, age...post hysterectomy side-effects perhaps?...

....Insidious is a great word, indeed, when describing the subtle changes that were taking place...First it was my face...which did not take on the super squaring or box look, but most definitely changed, and my features began morphing to the point that I no longer wished to appear in photos. I began to wonder who the stranger's face was that was staring back at me in the mirror....I knew this was not due to weight gain alone, for it was not a normal puffing, or fatty look, but an actual structural change....

....I had always had larger than normal size hands for a 5 ft. - 4 1/2 inch woman...but I began noticing that this too was increasing to the point where I could no longer buy rings that fit me....and if and when I allowed a photo to be taken, I was careful to find a way to hide what I began seeing as monstrous appendages, formerly known as hands...

....I eventually realized that something was happening to my feet and ankles as well....not so much in the length, but with an increase in the width and preponderance of hard tissue or bone growing on the top sides of my feet...This eventually made it almost impossible to buy shoes that fit...for even if the length and width accommodated my feet, I could not slide or slip the shoes over the tops of my feet....

....As for my ankles....both outer and inner....these also morphed... taking on a strange nuts and bolts look....then progressing to the point that it appeared that I had golf balls implanted beneath the skin on either side.....

....For someone who adored buying shoes and always considered herself to have quite lovely feet, it was a most painful and humiliating experience to shop for hours and days even, just to find a pair of shoes that fit properly....And of course this process was even more devastating when trying to find a pair of "dress" shoes....

...Other problems included, not finding a bra that fit well, due to the fact that my lower rib cage seemed to protrude unusually far, thus making the fit uncomfortable....or that "sexy" look pretty much an impossibility...I also developed many strange nodules or lumps under my skin...almost as if the tissue itself was changing....These fibrous nodules or tissue, which had at one time confined themselves to my breasts alone, now seemed to creep over my body, head to toe..

....In 2006, during a routine exam with my endocrinologist, it was discovered that I had nodules on my thyroid...after a suspicious biopsy, a complete thyroidectomy was in order...Following the thyroidectomy, results showed that indeed, I did have malignant thyroidal cancer...and therefore post-op, also received radio-active iodine therapy...

...For a short time, I was hopeful that all my strange symptoms were somehow thyroid related...but those hopes were soon dashed, as I realized that not only did they not improve, but continued to progress and increase...

...During that time, I underwent various other exams too; in lieu of the possibility of other health related issues, an MRI was performed. This exam just happened to pick up a small hypothalamic adenoma... As most adenomas of the pituitary system are considered benign, and no doctors picked up on any changes in my features...(more than likely due to the fact that they had never known the "old me")...I was sent on my way. This with only a passing mention that perhaps I should have another test run further down the road.

....Between that time, until the present day, visits to doctors have treated only symptoms. ....symptoms of pain...swelling....headaches... bi-polar disorder, and as you all well know...I could go on...and on......

.....Now, over the past few months, I have noticed that my headaches have been changing. Instead of the typical tension headache, or sinus related headache, I have been having episodes of severe, although brief, shooting or stabbing pain, over my left temple area. I have also had occasional pain in my left ear. At times I have heard a fluttering in both ears. I have experienced pain behind my left eye... a chronic twitch on the same side (which has actually been active for over 3 yrs. now)... seemingly rapid vision loss...and a bit of hearing loss as well.

....After recently mentioning the brief, left temple pain episodes to my doctor, she advised me that the next time I had such an episode I should head directly to the emergency room. She then added that she had the results from my MRI (which had been done while I was living overseas); it might be a good idea to take that to the hospital as well.

....Sure enough....this past Friday, it hit me once again! And off I went to the emergency room, MRI in hand. ...A warm and gentle doctor walked through the door that night, sat down in front of me, and began asking questions. He asked to see the MRI, and immediately mentioned the fact that I had an adenoma of one half a centimeter (considered micro), in my hypothalamus. ...

...But...amazingly, he did not stop there! He went on to ask me some very interesting questions...."Have you noticed any unusual changes in your body? ... Increase in size of feet for example?"...Well, as you can imagine, the flood gates opened, and out came everything that I had wanted to say to a doctor for so many years now. I told him that the only way I could describe what was happening to me is with a term my sister coined for these manifestations "the Neanderthal disease"....

....A CT was performed....showing indeed the existence of the adenoma. And the doctor then said the words "I have a name for your "Neanderthal disease," that name is "Acromegaly"...

....I have hope for the first time in my life....no health care coverage at present....but hope....

....Since returning stateside, I have not been able to acquire coverage, due to difficulty in finding employment. I have been receiving care through a clinic for people in my situation. One with limited resources. My unfortunate trip to the ER...well that will have to be worked out....I am now frantically in the process of finding a way to be accepted for Medicaid. As I do not qualify on the required terms, I must first go through Social Security Disability Assistance.

....One final note here....My release form from the ER, which required my signature, stated that I had read and understood my follow-up instructions:

#1- Go first thing in the morning to apply for Medicaid. ...

#2 Call a Dr. R. A., MD, Neurosurgery, for the soonest available appointment...

....So here I am... finishing this "story" in the wee hours of the morning....after the all-night exploration on all things Acromegaly, led me to you.....

.....I am only beginning this journey, which somehow feels like the end of a journey as well....

....To those of you who are still with me at these parting words...You are my heroes!!!

Author Unknown

I was really good at explaining away each and every issue that contributed to my appearance changing. I didn't call them symptoms because I didn't know I had anything. My hands developed arthritis and looked like they did because I did too much weed pulling in our yard. My feet grew because I gained 25 pounds and there was extra weight on them causing them to spread out. The weight contributed to my high blood pressure, snoring, and on and on. My age and a recent hysterectomy made me believe hormones might be involved in my skin changing, more facial hair and voice deepening, and my lack of libido.

So many chances to possibly detect it earlier. Every time I went to the dentist, I commented how my teeth had gone from a normal overbite to a serious under bite. I was clenching my teeth constantly, and the spaces between them had never been there before. I can remember never being able to floss comfortably and now I could probably floss an entire meal from in-between my teeth. Why didn't I question these changes?

Polyps were always found in my colonoscopies, each procedure finding more than the last time, and became more frequent. Kidney stones were plentiful in both of my kidneys.

I went to an ear, nose, and throat doctor for "Vertigo," but he didn't like the sound of my voice. He said it was too low and raspy. He asked me if my voice had changed, I said yes, and he proceeded with no advanced notice to look down my throat with a horrific tool; he found a polyp on my voice box. He booked me for a procedure, removed it, found that it was benign, but my voice didn't change.

My speech changed, the way words came out, but I really couldn't put my finger on it. A little mushy, a little slurring and a lot of beginning my sentences again. It felt like there was not enough room in my mouth for all of my teeth as well as my tongue.

None of these issues were life threatening, but very annoying and hard to understand why everything was changing.

By this time I had decided I had to lose weight, since I was carrying an extra 25 pounds. My arthritis was really bothering me, and it seemed to be in my back as well; and I had to get this under control. I joined weight watchers at our local parks and recreation gym. I lost 32 pounds in 8 months and was feeling good at least about one issue I was struggling with.

A very good friend was at the gym one day and pulled me aside to ask if I was okay; she had noticed that my tongue appeared large and swollen. I could not believe I needed someone else to tell me that. Why hadn't I noticed?

I saw a commercial that claimed a certain prescription might halt or slow down the progression of arthritis, and since my everyday tasks were becoming more difficult and more painful, I decided to go to a rheumatologist. I researched rheumatologists in the area, searching for a top doc and I found her, Dr. P. B., Rochester, Michigan.

She was the best.

I thought the exam would be as simple as sitting in an office with the doctor looking at my hands, maybe an x-ray or two and then handing me a prescription. Oh no....................All my clothes off, total examination. She asked me what seemed to be thousands of questions; I remember wondering why she had to know all this just because I have arthritis. When she asked about my hands changing in size, I said they had, and I had not been able to wear my wedding ring in at least 3 or 4 years. Then she asked about my feet, did they also hurt? I told her not at all, however I was hurt over the change in size because I could no longer wear cute shoes. I knew that she knew something was wrong.

She ordered loads of blood vials, and had many more questions. She told me she believed I had a disorder called "Acromegaly," and when the blood test results came back they would confirm it. She explained what Acromegaly was, but I swear I don't remember most of what she said. She referred me to a really great local endocrinologist who would see me the next week.

I drove home, raced to my computer and all I could remember was Acro and brain. Well of course that was enough to find out what I needed to know. I knew all the symptoms fit like a glove, but until the blood tests and MRI confirmed it, I didn't really believe it. It was too rare, or so they say.

My visit with the endocrinologist confirmed the Acromegaly diagnosis, and I cried all the way home. I had read enough to know that the first course of action was probably surgery.

All test results and MRI films were sent to the surgeon and in early July 2008, I gathered for the test results—it quickly filled up with my 2 doctors, 2 of my sisters, my husband, and finally me.

After all the details, and a lengthy explanation about Acromegaly, I was given a choice. I could choose surgery or I could opt to be part of a study titled: "Does Surgical Debulking of Pituitary Adenomas Improve Responsiveness to Octreotide-LAR in the treatment of Acromegaly; An Investigator-Initiated Study." I chose to be a part of a the study for 3 months prior to surgery. I needed time to get used to this and it seemed the right thing for me to do. I was given injections once a month and loads of blood work with each appointment. There was a possibility the tumor could shrink a little during this period.

By the end, my numbers had come down and the shots had been effective. I had transsphenoidal surgery on November 11th, 2008, and they were able to get 90% of the tumor, which was as predicted;

given the size of the tumor. I had a very short recovery time and by Christmas I was having parties and feeling just fine.

Also, as predicted, because the tumor was not completely removed, my January blood test showed high levels of GH and IGF, which means I have to have monthly injections the rest of my life. Thank God they have injections and thank God the injections work for me.

For me, the cosmetic issues of Acromegaly, rate as the hardest issue of the disorder for me to manage. I have never thought of myself as superficial, and I do not consider myself beautiful in the first place; however, when my looks got the best of my emotions, I got my doctor's blessing to deal with my issues more actively.

In July I had my nose reduced, and as I sit here getting my thoughts down on paper, my mouth is wired shut. I had jaw surgery 2 months ago. I'm starving, crabby and I haven't had anything that wasn't liquid in 8 weeks. Having said that, I would do it all over again, my top teeth are in front of my lower teeth, like they used to be, and a side benefit, I am almost at my goal weight.

I am grateful for:

- my endocrinologist for taking the time to explore the "total picture" of her patient, instead of just the apparent reason for that day's office visit.
- my surgeons. They are the VERY BEST.
- the fact that this disorder developed as an adult and not as a child.
- medicine being available that keeps my growth hormones normal.

David Terzo
Port Charlotte, FL

I was diagnosed with Acromegaly in May of 1999 and had my surgery to remove my pituitary tumor on June 23, 1999, in Gainesville,

Florida. But it was not that easy getting the diagnosis, at least for the several doctors that I had seen. I started having symptoms in the beginning of 1995, with just some tingling in my hands; it felt like my hands fell asleep, so I would sleep with my hands off the side of the bed so I could get the blood flowing again. If that did not work, I would just flick my fingers open and closed to push blood flow.

I was already going to see doctors regularly for a blood disorder called thalassemia minor, which is a form of anemia; a disease that resulted in my going for regular blood work. When the tingling would not stop, my doctor thought that it might have been related to the chemicals on the fruits and vegetables that I worked with, since I was a produce manager for our local food store. The doctor then suggested that I might also suffer from carpal tunnel syndrome and that I might need to have surgery to correct the problem, but I knew I was not willing to have that done. I have heard of too many people having problems after the surgery, so I just decided to wear a hand brace to alleviate the pressure on my wrists. This worked for a short time, but then I was suggested to see a chiropractor after my hands started to swell. The thought was that maybe something was wrong with the nerves in my hands or back, and that was affecting my hands. This went on for about a year before I decided to go see a Chinese doctor to try acupuncture treatments. After that, I tried massage to take care of possible nerve constrictions.

Those treatments lasted for about three years before I started having problems sleeping because I was snoring. I was snoring a lot! It was the family joke, and at times I would almost stop breathing until my wife Carolyn would shove me to wake up. This went on for several months. I was losing muscle tone, and I was not sure what was happening. As if all this was not enough, I also started having moments of extreme hot flash-like symptoms, and I noticed I was starting to get tired a lot more than normal.

Then one day we were out shopping, and a friend of ours that we had not seen in a while looked at me and said 'my gosh, what happened?' She noticed that my facial features were enlarged, but no one around me had noticed because they saw me every day. My tongue, nasal cavity, facial features, hands, and tongue were all enlarged. My hands and feet were also growing. I was growing so much that even my shoe sizes were changing. I tried different shoes and different brands, thinking that maybe they were made differently. I had wide feet. I was a 10½ EEE, and that was also my ring size. But almost before I knew it, I ended up with a 15½ EEE shoe size and a 15 ½ ring size.

We went to see an ear, nose, and throat doctor to see what was causing my snoring, and the doctor took one look at me and said that he thought that I might have something called Acromegaly. He sent me for blood work to confirm the diagnosis, and after the results came back, I was sent to an endocrinologist, where my wife and I would learn about this new disease.

Carolyn and I had just recently purchased our first home in 1998, and I had just been promoted to produce manager. Life was going great, and I was finally getting our life back on track. Then the appointment with the endocrinologist came. We sat in his office and with no compassion he said, "You have a brain tumor. You must resolve it or you will die in a year." I am not the type to really show emotions, but the tears rolled out, and I remember my wife saying that we are going to take care of this, I promise you. The doctor said that he did not know of any doctors who did the surgery and that I would have to research it on my own. We had just recently gotten a computer, so Carolyn researched Acromegaly and the different types of surgical procedures. We found a specialist who we became very fond of, and the time to surgery flew. I was diagnosed in May of 1999 and met with the neuro team in the second week of June. They offered to schedule the surgery for right after Independence Day, but I told them that I wanted the first available appointment, so I was scheduled for the very next week.

After the surgery, I had eight weeks of radiation therapy at a location about 3 ½ hours away from home. I could have had the radiation at a closer facility, but I trusted my doctor and was not willing to compromise. Because part of the tumor actually grew into my brain, I am still taking medication more than a decade later. I also need to take a testosterone replacement therapy to keep my testosterone where it should be. Lastly, I do make sure I get blood tests every three months, just to keep an eye on everything.

I am feeling great today. I got out of the retail business and got into the medical field, which I can only say happened because of the great care I received while in treatment for my Acromegaly. I wanted to give back as much as I received. My hands and feet went down in size a bit, and my facial features went back to somewhat normal, but as long as I wake up breathing, every day is a gift.

Fay Howard

Hi, my name is Fay Howard and I'm from Australia, married to a wonderful man now for almost 30 years with 2 sons aged 20 and 18.

Looking back, I guess my problems started with my thyroid operation in 1998 when a lump suddenly appeared in my throat that resulted in the removal of half of my thyroid. I didn't need any medication or anything, all seemed fine. That is, until 2004 when I went to my doctor complaining that I had been dropping things at work (night filling – restocking shelves at a local store). It seemed that I just couldn't keep a grip on things. And I would wake up in the morning with numbness in my hands and shooting pains up my arms. My general practitioner diagnosed me with Carpal Tunnel and referred me to a hand specialist who turned out to be my savior. I am so very grateful for his professionalism and thoroughness. I was just about through with my appointment with him, when I casually mentioned, maybe my rings would fit back on my fingers after the surgery. He looked at me and told me to sit back down. I told him I had had my rings resized twice in 24 years, and I thought I'd need them done again. With that, he sent me downstairs for an x-ray on my hands and told me to bring the pictures straight back to him; no need to get them reported. When I came back with the x-rays, he looked at them and said just as he thought! I didn't ask him what he meant, thinking it just confirmed the carpal tunnel. He said that I needed to make an appointment with my general practitioner as soon as possible. Apart from the carpal tunnel, I had no other symptoms of Acromegaly.

When I went to see my doctor, she almost literally dragged me into her office, saying that the specialist had rung her straight after my visit to fill her in. He thought that I was showing symptoms of a rare condition known as Acromegaly. She had gone home that night and read up on it as she said it was quite rare. The next thing she mentioned was the possibility of a brain tumor. Tears started to flow. What was happening? *One minute I have carpal tunnel, now you're telling me I might have a brain tumor?* My whole world was falling apart and I couldn't do anything to prevent it. I felt so useless.

My general practitioner put me in touch with a neurosurgeon, who immediately earned my faith and trust. He sent me for my first MRI; how scary are these things, I so hate them. My next step was to have a CT scan, and in fact I did have a pituitary tumor.

My hand surgery was scheduled and performed almost immediately. All went well with surgery, and I was given six weeks off of work to recover.

The day I was due to return to work from the carpal tunnel surgery was the day my neurosurgeon advised me that my transsphenoidal surgery had been scheduled and I would need 10 more weeks off work.

The day of my tumor surgery came and my husband and sons drove me to the hospital. When we arrived they were told they couldn't stay with me in the waiting area, as there wasn't that much room. They were told to just go home. My surgery was delayed anyway because the previous patient had run over time in surgery. I was left to sit and worry by myself for hours before I was finally prepped for surgery.

I didn't know what time it was, but when the nurse woke me in the recovery room and I opened my eyes my husband and 2 sons were there. They told me it was after midnight; my neurosurgeon had rung them to let them know my surgery had gone well but there had been a delay, which was why it was so late. They said that they didn't care, they just wanted to see me. My husband later told me that when they were told to leave the hospital before surgery, he didn't know if he would see me again.

The first thing I was aware of was that I had dried blood on both sides of my head and also this headache, it was like something was squeezing my head. The surgeon told me that was the brace they had to use to hold my head in place during surgery, and the packing in my nose, while a little uncomfortable, had to remain in for five days.

After surgery, I was introduced to another doctor; an endocrinologist. I was told she would monitor my levels. I was healing nicely. The pressure headaches weren't as bad, and the nose packing could be removed, so I was released from hospital and told to take it easy.

My neurosurgeon thought he had removed all the tumor; unfortunately an after-scan proved there was still some residual tumor and it appeared to be wrapped around a blood vessel, so further surgery was not an option. I went to see the endocrinologist, and she said that my levels had dropped but not enough, so my journey with prescription medication began.

Before I could start on the shot, I had an ultrasound done on my gallbladder that revealed I had a small polyp that the injections could irritate, making things harder to treat. So the doctors decided to just remove my gallbladder. After surgery I would start on my monthly injections. The nursing staff at the hospital that administer these to me each month are so lovely; they all feel for me and my horse needle that is as blunt as anything.

Four years after surgery, in September 2008, I had an MRI checkup. It showed no sign of any residual tumor. My neurosurgeon asked me if I had had any radiotherapy, and I said no. He then asked me if I had thought about the Gamma Knife surgery we discussed. I said no, but I had to ask why. He said that "pathology is at a loss for the MRI because there is no sign of the residual tumor." When I heard that, I remembered that I had an endocrinologist's appointment on Thursday, October16, and I was hoping that my shot dosage would be lowered, due to this news.

Now, five years removed from the start of my journey, my latest MRI still shows no sign of any residual tumor or any new growth. My neurosurgeon wonders how long he needs to send me for MRIs, but I don't have to see him for 18 months now. They have lowered my injections to every six weeks now, but kept the dosage the same.

Overall I feel fine. My life is almost the way it was before all of my surgeries. The only difference is that I still get tired and depressed more often. When I do struggle with this, I read about someone else's ordeals with Acromegaly and I realize that I'm not alone; there are other people that understand what I feel, and that helps.

I'm one lucky lady. I have very caring medical professionals looking after me, and my family have always been very loving and supportive. Because of my sons' ages, I think they were able to handle things better than if they had been littlies.

This letter was written from an Acromegalic struggling with the disease, and with a close friend. Names have been changed to protect all parties involved, but there is a lesson to be learned from this letter. Acromegaly is very difficult to cope with, both for the patient, and for the people who love them.

Name intentionally Withheld

February 10, 2009

Dear Friend,

I hope you are doing well. I cannot believe it has been over three months or more that we have not really talked. Although I can fill the time easily I know I can never replace the friendship that I had with you. I miss it tremendously.

I want you to know what has gone on since we last talked. The night you called and mentioned that you were concerned, I was a mess. I ended up in the ER the same night with an extreme panic attack. I have never told you or anyone else this because it is what it is. I basically had hit rock bottom. I had just lost one of the best friends I had here in town. My question though I had not answered was WHY?

I have been struggling over the past months with this question. I still do not have an answer but this is how I see it:

Anna was being nasty, as you put it. She was not being nice to John and would not ride in your car without a major fight. Why was she doing this? Was it her fault?

NO. It was clearly mine.

I was on many medications, under the guidance of my doctors. I was in the middle of changing medications, as I was constantly. I was not able at the time to be consistent with ANNA. I let things that meant little to me at the time slide. (ONE major one being that I should have IMMEDIATELY corrected her when she was not nice to John.)

Looking back, I know I should have done this but I did not and I was truly doing the best that I could do.

Secondly, I want you to know that I do appreciate you expressing your concerns about my medications. That I was on medications that you did not feel I needed. That I had depression but no longer seemed depressed. AS I mentioned before I cannot tell you how much I would LOVE to be off of EVERY ONE of my medications. However I am still on a medication called "S" and this medication cuts off my growth hormone so it does not get high again. It also cuts off other hormones too. These hormones cannot all just be replaced by exercising enough, thinking happy thoughts, or praying. Trust me I soooo wish they could. It has been VERY VERY hard for me to accept the fact that I might have to be on these medicines for the rest of my life. However, I have lifted up all my fears to God and know I am in his hands. I make the best INFORMED decision I have each and every time I have to make one.

I sit here and type and wonder if I should even send this to you. Will it begin to repair our friendship? I hope it does and pray you hear what I am trying to say to you. I am sorry if I have hurt you in any way. I am sorry if I was not the friend to you that you needed (the friend to go with you to the zoo, the friend to work out consistently with you, the friend to listen) I know I have been the friend to take over the years and not the friend who was giving. I am and will always be thankful for all that you gave me. You gave me hours of free counseling, personal training, personal organizing, and always came to lend me a hand even when I did not ask. You have always been there for me. I just want you to know that I am thankful and will always be here to give back to you in any way that I can give back.

Again I am sorry if I hurt you in any way. I am sorry if Anna hurt John.

I know God Closes Doors and Opens Windows. I really think that all of this was in his plan. I just wish he would have left out our friendship coming to an end.

I have been working hard over the last three months to become the best mother and friend that I can be. I now have Anna in a pre-school and I am able to take her to school and pick her up myself without relying on others to help me. I have also been working on my health and am in the best possible place I can be. I pray that you read this and understand that I really am sorry. Coming up to your door with the note saying our friendship was over was hateful, impulsive and mean. Please forgive me.

I know this may sound silly but I really do love you and your family too. I wish you all the best. You have all taught me many many lessons in life.

Sincerely,

Alecia E

When I think about Acromegaly, the two people that I immediately think of are André the Giant and Richard Kiel, famous for his role as "Jaws" in 007. After I was diagnosed, I searched the internet for more information or pictures of non-famous people who had the disease—hoping to find images of women with Acromegaly. But there was not much I could find. What I did find were mounds and mounds of repeat information defining Acromegaly and how to treat it. Surely there's got to be someone else out there that is keeping a journal about this!

I kept asking myself, "What will I look like?"

I continued searching...

Everything I read only confirmed the physical changes I was already experiencing. I had symptoms relating to both prolactinoma and Acromegaly. A few of those problems included the fact that my facial skin began to thicken, and pimples were breaking out more frequently than the once in a while I was used to. I also continued to lactate after my youngest daughter was weaned for two years, I began to sweat a lot and had horrible headaches. The headaches were in a category of their own. I cannot really describe them to you other than to say that the pressure was unbearably skull-splitting, and it was hard to tell where they originated. The headaches would come over me seemingly instantaneously; they had no pattern, except that they did seem to happen more at night. As time went on these headaches became more frequent and longer lasting. Worst of all, they started to happen at any time of the day. Usually when I felt a headache coming on, the intense pain washed over me within minutes.

I began having headaches shortly after we moved from California to Texas in 1999. I had no history of headaches and so a CT scan was ordered by my general practitioner. Test results came back as "normal." At this point my doctor assumed, and I believed, that the headaches were allergy-related because of the fact that this all started after our move to an area where bad allergy problems were common. I never really pursued another answer for the headaches after that, although I mentioned it whenever I went to the doctors. I frequently took naproxen sodium whenever I had a headache—this made me tired enough to eventually drift off to sleep.

In addition to the other symptoms I had, I developed chronic pain in my left ear. For almost two years I visited several doctors including two ear, nose, and throat doctors and a TMJ physician to find the cause. The TMJ physician ran tests, and told me that I didn't have TMJ. The ENT doctor, who referred me to the TMJ doc, insisted I had a real problem, despite what was told to him. I asked if he could order an x-ray or something to look deeper in my ear, but he felt there was no justification for it because I had a "classic case" of TMJ. He didn't think it was necessary to look any further until I went back to the TMJ doctor for *more* testing. I decided to get yet *another* opinion from a third ENT who ordered an MRI and found the tumor. When this ENT broke the news to me he said that my inner ear "looked great" but that I had a giant tumor in the middle of my head. He referred me to a neurosurgeon for further treatment.

This is an excerpt from a letter between friends. All key information has been deleted to protect all parties, but it is a great example of how a patient can feel overwhelmed by the medical universe.

Author Intentionally Withheld

Dear ____:

I just wanted to be clear that "doctor shopping" is a negative thing, and that I do not doctor shop! Actually this is a VERY VERY fine line.

For 23 years I went to the same doctors, then the __ health center maybe a time or two.

Then age 23 to age 30 ONLY went to Dr. R. Yes, starting at age 30 I realized that getting second opinions is 100% necessary.

I trusted B. What happened, the other doctor put me on too much medication that raised my sodium levels to the point that they almost killed me. (Dr. D realized this although it is not noted in my file like this.)

Second, S put me on Estrogen. Made me sick. S put me on Bromocroptine. This medicine only works sometimes. He did say he used it because it was easier to administer and less expensive, and after I asked him about Sandostatin LAR he then said he would change me to it if I would like. At this point I went to Mass General to get a second opinion (or doctor shop if you would like to call it that). Since I did that, they if you remember, started me on the Sandostatin there and I did not have to take the daily injections. They were the best. Yes I wanted the best.

When I came back I needed someone here to take care of me. Found V. Has it been a perfect fit? NO. Does B have a better endo? NO. The best endos for ME that deal specifically with my issues are spread across five states, and my home state is not one of them. This is okay but I would prefer working with an endo that actually goes to meetings held by recognized pituitary associations.

Next Primary Care. D is great. However he is far [distance]. They do blood work in their office and the nurses are terrible at taking blood because they use larger needles, I think that they are less expensive. If he was closer and not your friend would I have stayed with him? YES.

Next, yes I have been sent to doctors for everything from my colon to my kidneys....my primary will not do all this herself. Does this make it complicated? Yes. Do I wish I could go to ONE doctor only? YES. Am I always looking for someone who can care for ALL of me? YES.

Next my psychiatrist. My friend suggested I see one. D said it was a good idea. I was only going to go once. As you know I am still seeing Dr. H as my primary physician. Are my medicines causing me problems right now? I would guess yes. Is Dr. H trying to get me off of them or back to a point I can make it through the day without sleeping? Yes. Have I asked my primary to just handle my psychiatrist meds? Yes. What did she say? NO. Could I go to another psychiatrist and save money? YES. Am I willing to do this? NO. Why? I have spent almost six years with Dr. H. I have full trust in her that she is going to get me off of these medicines. Then she will be there if I need help again. She is the ONLY doctor I know that will let me leave messages for HER. She checks them (not staff) and SHE calls me back. I ONLY DEAL with ONE person. HER. So she knows everything. It is a security to me as other offices it is like a phone chain before getting a message from the doctor and you do not hear back from the doctor.

Now that I think about it though....D....did call me back himself EVERY TIME....

Dr. R, my primary I do like. She is VERY smart but has three young children. I have no plans to change any of the following doctors ever, unless we move. Although I do not like to be dependent on anyone but myself, I am dependent on them at this point.

My goal for the year was to get off any medicine I did not need.

I am now only on Sandostatin 10mg every two months.

I am completely off all ADD medicines.

I am only on 5mg of Lexapro.

I am on a middle dose, pretty high for me, of Wellbutrin 300mg.

And am on the Singulair now for allergies.

I have been off the Ativan for 9 months! I am going to get thought my MRI in June without taking it. Not sure how, but I will just pray a lot I guess.

I am off the high doses of Lexapro.

What was causing all my heart problems and my waking up in the middle of the night, fainting, and then going stiff....no one knows. I KNOW though it was not in my head. It had to be my medicines.

It has basically been a year and a half of hell. My hormones are high and low and we have been trying to find the right dose of Sandostatin. For a few months it was too high. For a few months too low. It is just a guessing game really.

When I first get the shot for a few weeks I seem to get low blood sugar and get really cold. Before my period starts I get really hot, swollen and moody too.

Have I "shopped" around to get all this information? YES. Is it a negative thing? NO.

A lady at a local store, who is very sweet, told me she and her husband got divorced this past year because he was addicted to prescription drugs. Specifically, Ativan. Went to a few centers for treatment but I guess it did not work. She made the comment that he would "doctor shop." This just really hit a nerve with me because when you are SICK even if it is sickness "addiction" you are going to shop around for a doctor to help you. It is NEVER the patient's problem; it is the doctor's problem. Patients should NOT be scared or feel guilty for getting second or third opinions. Doctors should know what they are doing and follow up with patients. Not just give them medicine and then ONLY see them if they decide to come back. If a doctor gives a patient medicine it should be the responsibility of that doctor [to] follow through....a sick person is someone that needs someone watching out for them.

Ok off my soap box for now. I hope I got my point across.

The following is a collection of blog excerpts printed with permission from Alecia E. from http://blessed-beyondmeasure.blogspot.com

Acceptance

It was not suspected right away that I had acromegaly once the tumor was found. I first met with a neurosurgeon in Dallas who, fortunately, did not look at me and right away say, "there sits a gal with acromegaly." As a matter of fact, he didn't order blood work to rule the disease out because he was convinced my tumor was not acromegalic. I didn't LOOK like I had acromegaly because I am 5' 2" and do not have giant extremities or the typical acromegaly appearance. The changes have been subtle and slow. Given another ten years (without the tumor being discovered) it might have been the case that I looked really different.

I was told that if the tumor was not found, I would have likely gone blind or had obvious visual disturbances which would have [led] to the discovery eventually. Had it not been for the persistence of my ENT to find the cause of ear pain, which may have been my story. Once I was referred to an endocrinologist, he began to look at little deeper at the possibility of acromegaly. David and I knew before I had the surgery that this was most likely my diagnosis.

I cannot tell you how, as a woman, it feels to look at Richard Kiel, Jaws in James Bond, and the person who has always scared the crud out of me, and find out we share the same disease. I wondered if those were now going to be my most prominent features. Would my face begin to take on a more masculine and coarse shape? Would my hands and feet continue to grow and become really huge? I began to look in the mirror and wonder what I would look like in a few years. I thought the changes that I was experiencing were a normal process of aging. I had no idea a brain tumor could transform a person's appearance. It was becoming a reality for me and I had to accept that I was sick - it was a hard thing to accept.

Hours before Surgery

The night before my brain (pituitary) tumor was removed, my husband and I went to dinner alone at our old-time favorite restaurant. Then, after dinner we made a quick stop at my parents' house to kiss them goodbye, Dave and I left for UCLA. We reserved a room to stay near the UCLA Medical Center campus. Since my surgery was first thing in the morning, we thought it would be easier to be close-by and not deal with the traffic.

It was a long night. Dave and I tried to sleep but couldn't and didn't. We watched the clock count down every minute. I took a shower, trying to calm my nerves. The light against the stark white bathroom walls was unnerving. I kept thinking about God and wondered what my life would be like in 24 hours...what the outcome of the surgery would be. I thought about my kids. I missed them...I prayed, I cried, and I prayed some more. I was scared. Dave was too. After I got out of the shower, I just lay in bed waiting for the alarm to go off; reminding me I needed to leave for the hospital.

We arrived at the hospital and went through the routine paperwork. I had to give a copy of my living will. Dave and I had our wills written about two months prior to the discovery of the tumor. Good thing I planned ahead...I had no idea I'd be using mine so soon. After everything was completed I waited to be called to the operating room. When I was called back for the operation, the nurse offered some medicine to help take the edge of my nerves while inserting the IV. I accepted the offer because I NEEDED it! Before I drifted off my husband said "you mentioned that if you didn't make it out of the operation to tell the family hi for me and to read, *Just in Case You Ever Wonder* (by Max Lucado) to the kids. I fell asleep before I could utter the words, "I love you..."

Waking up from Surgery

The first thing I recall while waking up from surgery was Dr. Kelly's wide, black-rimmed glasses looking at my face very close up. "Can you see me...Alecia, can you see? How are you doing...can you see?" There was concern that I could lose my sight during the operation. The tumor had grown against my optic nerve so there was a chance that I would not have my sight when I awoke. I gave Dr. Kelly a thumbs-up and nod because that's about all I could do. My mind was working normally but I was still so drugged up I couldn't communicate very well. I had a lot of questions. I tried to make sense of the sensations I had physically post surgery. My lungs were heavy, my wrist hurt (where they put an arterial gas line), the roof of my mouth was numb. Thoughts continued to race through my mind - *I'm alive...I can see. Did I lose my pituitary? Am I okay?* I continued to observe the discussions of the doctors and nurses around me hoping to hear answers to the questions I had.

They removed my tumor by going through my nose. Dr. Kelly removed the bone from my sphenoid sinus, cutting through the skull base and then through the dura (brain lining). He does NOT pack the sinuses after surgery, but only tapes thick gauze across the bottom of the nose. The only complication I had (if it could be called that) was a mild CSF (cerebral spinal fluid) leak during the operation. It was repaired with a titanium mesh and collagen sponges. The tumor was both gelatinous and fibrous in nature. As Dr. Kelly got closer to my pituitary, the tumor was more fibrous making it a challenge to spare the gland. He began slicing micro-layers of the tumor away until normal pituitary gland was found via pathology exam. I didn't lose my gland. Dr. Kelly managed [to] save it! I barely took any pain medicine post surgery. Some of the discomfort I experienced was a numb palate and drippy/stuffy nose. I lost my sense of smell (completely) for a couple weeks but it eventually returned. I still have very mild numbness/tingling on the front part of my palate but I am used to it now. Up to this day (15 months post surgery) I have NO DAMAGE to my pituitary gland and endocrine functions are all normal.

Part of the tumor was deemed "inoperable" because it had grown into the cavernous sinus which harbors the carotid artery so my neurosurgeon said any attempt to remove it would be catastrophic. It was possible, but not likely, that the tumor could fall out of that area while the rest was being removed. Thank God, the unlikely happened and a majority, if not all, [of] the tumor came out of the cavernous sinus.

Feeding Baby Post-Surgery

A couple weeks after getting home and settled, I started getting concerned about my daughter's weight. She seemed awfully small compared to what my other three children weighed at her age. I began weighing her on the scale at home and noticed she wasn't gaining weight since her 4 month check up in June. I went digging through my children's baby books to see what their weight was at 6 months. All of them had more than doubled their weight and were above 16 pounds. Danielle was barely 13 pounds (she weighed 8 lbs 4 oz in February). I began to suspect my milk production was diminishing.

I took Danielle in for her 6 month check up last week and although she was doing well, her weight is in the 5% range (13 pounds 11 ounces). My suspicions were confirmed - she was under weight. Her little growth curve has taken a downward turn. I asked the pediatrician if he thought maybe she wasn't getting enough breast milk and he said it was possible given my history of pituitary surgery; however, he was not too concerned because my daughter's length and head circumference is growing nicely. He recommended I try to up my milk production using Fenugreek, an ancient herb that aids in milk production; but he suggested I ask my doctor first because of my medical history. Fenugreek spurs on prolactin and the pituitary tumor I had produced both a prolactin and growth hormone, so he wasn't sure it was safe for me.

When I got home I tried expressing milk during feeding time to see how much milk I was producing and I could barely get an ounce! This is very abnormal for me. I called my doctor and told him what was going on and wanted to see if there was any way to know whether something was wrong with my pituitary function and he said no. He said I cannot take Fenugreek or anything that would help with milk production because it might spur on tumor growth. He advised I supplement since there is suspicion of milk depletion. This was strange to me. I fed all three of my other kids with ease for at least a year. Although, I had wondered if there would be an issue breastfeeding Danielle post-pituitary surgery, I had no problems right after I delivered her. In her first few months, she was thriving, so there was no question as to whether I could breastfeed successfully. Now it appears I was not producing enough milk. In light of the situation, I had to have to supplement and see if it helped with Danielle's weight gain.

Dealing with Emotions

My step-dad told me he was amazed at how strong I appeared on the outside during this whole ordeal before the surgery and afterwards. He said he knew I just had to be very scared inside... he was right. When I first heard about the tumor I was completely numb. The fear that went through me is indescribable. Saying I was shocked would be an understatement. For the most part I tried to stay calm but when I really sat a while and thought about what I was facing, I cried uncontrollably. There were many nights when my husband joined me in the tears.

When I came out of surgery I'm not sure I was prepared for the emotions that followed. Feelings of bitterness and despair surfaced. I got home from the hospital a day earlier than expected because my recovery was so remarkable. Instead of staying in the hospital the expected 3-4 days I was released from UCLA on the morning of the second day (I had surgery on Friday morning and went home Sunday morning). I was glad my recovery was going well, but frustrated about what I was going through. Inside I was grumbling about the fate that had been given me. The anger I had was very strange, not like anything I'd ever had before.

The feelings began when I was in the hospital. I was irritated at the catheter they put in me as well as the machines and wires around me. I felt trapped. My level of discomfort was minimal, but waiting to hear if my pituitary was okay was stressful. It required a lot of patience. Recovery also required patience. Any life altering physiological changes as a result of the surgery were still unknown. Everything was uncertain and all the routine stability I had in my life was missing. My life had turned upside down. Although I was exhausted emotionally I tried to be mindful of the others who were helping. Trying not to complain was challenging, but I did my best.

After the surgery I had a lot of quiet time to recover, as we lived with my parents for three weeks. You would think that I would have enjoyed the quiet time and use it to rest but I couldn't. I felt very alone, scared, and angry. No one was near if I needed help - no one. My parents were understandably busy with their schedules, and everyone went [on] with their normal routines...except me. I sat alone in the house, bleeding out the nose, a hole drilled in my head, and tried to make sense of the circumstances I found myself in. I felt abandoned even though I knew I hadn't been. I just didn't want to be alone. In desperation, that evening I called my mom and asked her to pick me up from my in-laws. She and my sister took me to a nearby coffee shop. I tried to keep my chin up, but it was hard to. It was nice to get out of the house. I wanted to get out - even if it was just to sit somewhere, because I wanted to be okay like everyone else.

I can't really put my finger on any one thing that made me upset, just that I was. I dealt with this in my own way, by just trying to ignore my feelings and act contrary to how I felt. In reality this was probably the best thing for me to do at the time. I might have lashed out and said things I didn't mean. I'm certain I am not alone when I speak of the loneliness and anger I felt when going through this. From the beginning I accepted my fate but once it became a reality and the surgery was done - I grew impatient waiting for the results. Something I wasn't keeping in mind was that my husband's world was upside down as well. Although he didn't go through the surgery, he was feeling the effects of it too. He just didn't have time to show it. We were thousands of miles away from our home, stuffed in someone else's house with our three kids and trying to maintain normalcy. Everyone that helped out devoted their time willingly, and their lives were interrupted too. Before the surgery I was determined to make the best of the situation and remain upbeat but I had no idea how difficult that would be...accepting this change of life was not easy. At times I was bitter even though I went through it with a smile.

The anger disappeared as days went by. With each doctor visit I received good news that the surgery may have been successful. After a few weeks, life got completely back to normal and I wasn't mad at the world anymore. I chose to not stay mad, although I did find myself still battling to accept my uncertain future with contentment. Maybe a lot of the anger had to do with hormones and changes that occurred as the pituitary dropped back into place? I don't know... but I doubt it!

Coping with Good Days and Bad Days

Jaki Loebig

But they that wait upon the Lord shall renew their strength; they shall mount up with wings as eagles; they shall run, and not be weary; and they shall walk, and not faint.

—Isaiah 40:31

From my earliest memories, life was filled with all sorts of challenges. My birth mother disappeared from my life when I was three years old, after months of my parents playing "snatch and grab" with me and my younger brother. We didn't know where we were half the time. My birth mother was so frightened of my father's violence that she would take us and hide with us in halfway houses, or anywhere that she could find refuge. Regardless, my father always found us, and after a lot of shouting would drag us back to his home. It was a dreadful time for my family.

My father gained custody over us when I was five years old, mostly because at the time of the court hearing, my brother and I were in his possession. The social worker said we'd been moved around so much it would be harmful for us to be moved again.

My mother married another man only a few months after her divorce, despite him being a known pedophile. He had his own business and was very comfortable financially, and I'm sure this would have been her motivation. My father told me that my mother didn't want me, didn't love me, never wanted to see me again, and that I was to never ever ask for her. My brother didn't speak for months afterward. If I am hurt, I let people know what the problem is, rather than let it fester, and this was reflected by my behaviour at the time. From then on I felt like I was a reject. My mother didn't want me, and my father had no idea at all on how to be a good parent. He would lose his temper, shouting threats like: "I'll knock you into the middle of next week"; "I'll crown you and it won't be king"; "I'll give you something to cry for"; then wallop me really hard. Sometimes, after the anger diminished, he would regret his violence, apologize, and cuddle me.

While my mother married someone of questionable values, my father didn't do much better. He had several lady friends, all women with their own families already, so my brother and I would be dragged along, unwelcome additions to liaisons in their own homes. He had no discretion about what he was doing, and I saw him having sex on more than one occasion. None of these relationships lasted very long. I grew up emotionally confused. It seemed to me that sex and/or violence were necessary ways to get affection.

School Days

I found it difficult to make friends when I started school because I was the only child in the school without a mother. Moreover, by the time I got to school, my father had been diagnosed with multiple sclerosis and was unable to work, so we lived in dire poverty.

When I was ten years old, my father married again. He told me that if I ever upset my stepmother he would put me in a children's home. I am confident that he meant it too. In an ironic twist, my father and his second wife became born-again Christians just before they married. Unfortunately, though, this did nothing to help my father's foul temper and violent nature. And after they were married, they also had children of their own; another boy and girl—so my brother and I were again marginalized like a modern version of Cinderella, not quite getting the leftovers, but the message was clear that HER kids came first. When I changed schools at age 11, I went to a school for the bright children. Unfortunately for me though, I was the only working class kid among my peers. My parents couldn't afford the proper uniform or sports equipment. I felt like I wore my poverty on my back for all to see, suffering the shame of free school meals and walking part of the way to school because my stepmother wouldn't pay the whole bus fare. I wasn't picked on at school, but I think it is simply because bullying didn't happen in my school. That being said, I was certainly ostracised for being different. Throughout my childhood, I remember being cold and hungry, not only for food and shelter, but equally for love, affection, and support.

I was forced to attend church every Sunday, where the message I heard was the same one that I got at home: that I was condemned to Hell as a sinner, reinforcing my belief that I was a reject. I left school at 17 years old, with the equivalent of good High School grades and secretarial qualifications. My goal was clear in my mind: get a job and escape from the poverty.

When I was 17, I finished high school and got a job. Now I was desperately looking for love. At the time I had been having a secret relationship with a man fourteen years older than me. He was an absolute charmer. I was fourteen the first time he kissed me, fifteen when I started seeing him, and barely sixteen when he took my virginity. My stepmother found out about our relationship and went into such a deep sulk that my father ordered me to pack my bags and go. I moved in with my lover, and three months later we were married. Because of my youth and naiveté, I didn't realize that it was only lust, and not love that he felt for me. As I began to realize this, I felt like I had jumped out of the frying pan and into the fire. I think he must have married only because circumstances conspired against him, plus because of the pressure from my family.

First Awareness of Acromegalic Symptoms

I had symptoms of Acromegaly throughout my adolescence, without even realizing what was going on. I had my first severe headache at thirteen, a headache that actually had me laid up in bed for a week. The doctor said it was migraine and gave me painkillers. As I grew older, these headaches became more frequent. I assumed the headaches were a by-product of my lifestyle, since I was always awake late into the night listening to pirate radio stations. As I grew older, my lifestyle did not improve that much. Radio was not my biggest problem anymore; I frequently drank too much alcohol, smoked about thirty cigarettes a day, and partied all night. Always one to take his shot at me, my father told me on multiple occasions that I would be a slut just like my birth mother, so I guess I had something to live up (or down) to. I would later discover that these headaches, which would regularly lay me flat for two or three days, were in fact a tumor manifesting its presence.

From the time I was a young child, I chewed my nails down to the quick, leading my stepmother to constantly remind me that I would have stubs instead of fingertips, which led me to just ignore fingertips altogether. Maybe if I had paid more attention to my fingers, I would have noticed the massive growth in my hands. Since one of the symptoms of Acromegaly is growth of the hands and feet, I figure that her ridiculing me led to me missing another warning sign.

And sweat! Did my feet sweat! The salt would come through the surface of my leather shoes, causing them to disintegrate prematurely, once again providing a joke for the family at my expense. I was told I had inherited this trait from my birth mother. By the time I hit my early twenties, my palms had joined with my sweaty feet in that they were often home to puddles of perspiration.

Even my eyes would give me trouble. As I grew into my adolescence, my eyes grew very light-sensitive, apparently quite common in acromegalics. It would actually hurt when my pupils contracted in response to bright light, so I had to purchase my first pair of polarised sunglasses at the young age of seventeen. They cost me £8.00 [about $13], half of my weekly wage back then. I always wore sunglasses whenever the sun poked its head out from behind the clouds, and I still have to today.

Adulthood

When I was 18 years old, I was five feet six inches, but two years later when I was about to deliver my first child, I discovered that I had gained another half inch. My recent growth spurts would become most clear to me when I was at home one day combing my hair while my husband was having a shave. All of a sudden, it seemed, I was taller than him even though we had been the same height when we married. He was very insecure about his height, so he accused me of standing on my tiptoes just to humiliate him. That prompted me to measure myself, and I discovered that I had gained a further 2½ inches since having my son, five years previously. When I was 24 and at the maternity clinic again, and they measured me, I had grown *another* inch taller *again*. When I pointed this out to the nurse, she told me not to be stupid; that could not possibly be the case. In fact, by the time I would finally be diagnosed, I would have grown to be 5'10" tall. While it would be easy to blame my disease on a medical oversight of my doctors, even when I was working at medical offices, signs and symptoms were missed.

As I was growing as an adult I had terrible pains in the long bones in my legs. They felt like growing pains, but I figured that was impossible since I was in my twenties and finished growing. I wanted to talk to my doctor, but I could only imagine how he would have reacted if I told him I was suffering from growing pains! Anyhow, I was too frightened to see my doctor about this because I feared what it might really be. My father was one of eight children; and since my father and three other siblings had Multiple Sclerosis, I was afraid that would be my diagnosis as well. As a child I was told that MS was not a genetic disorder, but it just seemed too realistic a possibility with all of my aches. I told a friend that I felt like something was wrong with me, but I couldn't put my finger on it, and I just hoped that I would figure out what was wrong before it killed me.

I noticed that my face was changing, which made no sense. I thought I must be losing my marbles since faces don't change, except to get older and wrinkly! My lips began to look like I'd had botox injections, and my nose was growing longer. My cheek bones widened, becoming more prominent. My bottom jaw was growing, my face changed from a heart-shape to more of a square. I was getting gaps between my teeth that, if I had not already stopped biting my nails, I would have had to because my teeth would not meet. I covered my heavy brow with a full fringe. My hair was also becoming very thick and wiry.

It seemed like my frame was also growing. The buttons on a dress that used to fit me well, all of a sudden, would refuse to meet over my rib cage. Not only that, but I had a beautiful full-length fitted leather coat I loved to wear that I had to give away because I could not do the buttons up. The zippers on my jeans were pulling apart in the middle. While I had a flat stomach, my hip bones were growing. I knew I was not getting fat; it's just that my rib cage was growing, which made no sense to me.

Beyond my midsection, my shoe size had gone up three sizes in ten years, and my hands became big, to match the rest of me. Before I knew it, I was wearing men's large-size gloves. Even when I want to wear a hat, I have found it impossible to get a ladies' hat to fit my oversized head, so I either make the hats myself or I have to wear a man's fedora.

Maybe all of these symptoms should have been noticed, but I was so busy raising my children and working to take much notice of what was happening to me, physically.

Me and My Disease

Early symptoms of Acromegaly were easily missed. When I would complain to my doctor that I didn't feel right, I was dismissed. When I was in my early thirties, I was very tired all the time – deep down 100% exhausted, tired enough to actually discuss it with the doctor. My General Practitioner said: "You've got 2 children and a full time job – how do you expect to feel?" On top of that, since I had grown up with my father's MS, I compared all of my problems to that, and anything that had happened to me seemed insignificant.

Even as a young girl when I was eleven, I have always endured abnormally heavy menstruations. It was in pursuit of reasons for my problem that would eventually result in the discovery of my pituitary tumor. I was sent to a gynecologist at a hospital in London. This hospital is part of a teaching hospital, so I was initially interviewed by a medical student who asked a lot of questions. I told him I thought I was still growing, and he looked a bit surprised. I saw the consultant who glared at me over his half glasses and asked me what other illnesses I had suffered. I was sure that he suspected me of having Munchausen's, but when I told him I had had glandular fever when I was thirteen years old, plus two healthy pregnancies, he began to take proper notice of what might be the underlying cause of my problems.

I was referred to the endocrinologist where I was given a glucose tolerance test, which made me very sleepy. He gave me a blood test which revealed my thyroid gland was getting no instruction from the non-existent pituitary. No surprise there. I continually complained about being tired until my dosage of thyroxine was increased from 100 mcg to 300 mcg. It took frequent visits over about eighteen months, without pre-arranged appointments to the consultant's clinic, to achieve this increase in dosage. He was very kind, always saw me when I turned up and listened to what I had to say. It turns out that I produced far too much insulin in response to sugar, so they did it again another day and the same thing happened. The test showed abnormally high levels of growth hormone and I was sent for a CT scan, which found the tumor.

It was October 1982 when I was finally diagnosed with Acromegaly, at 28 years old. I would have the surgery four months later, in January 1983. The delay was to run other tests to make sure that my internal organs were not enlarged. When they did the surgery, it took the surgeon four hours just to saw through the thickened bones of my nose. After surgery I was informed by the surgeon that they were 99.9% sure they had cut out the entire tumour. Muscle was cut from the top of my leg to use as a patch under my brain. I had fifteen yards of bandages packing out my sinuses for ten days. I will never forget the headache. I was given a sedative before the bandages were removed—my request for a glass of brandy was sadly refused! The surgeon told me not to blow my nose for three weeks or I would be blowing out brain matter! I was put on steroids for a few weeks in case my hypothalamus went into shock.

I had six monthly visits to the endocrinologist for the first 3 years after surgery, and then annual checkups with blood tests to keep an eye on my hormone levels. Only a year after surgery, a routine CT scan would show tumour remnants were growing again, and so was the rest of me.

Almost immediately after the discovery of tumor remnants, I began daily radiation treatments, every weekday morning for a month. After a month, a new CT scan showed the tumour and the remains of the pituitary had been destroyed. I was thrilled about that, but now I had to put my visible life back together. My hair fell out around the irradiated areas on both sides of my head; it eventually grew back but baby fine. The radiation did not burn me, but I think that is because I still had skin like cowhide. The ducts that drain fluid from my eyes were inflamed. I had tinnitus for weeks – it sounded like a Wurlitzer piano had moved into my head, playing random chords day and night.

The Psychological Side of a Physical Struggle

The psychological effects of my physical changes were never considered by any of the medical professionals. After I was diagnosed, my then-husband (now ex-) was very unkind about my physical changes. He would frequently call me a freak or an Amazon. He would also rant about having to put up with my emotional needs—in fact he told me if I wanted emotional support to go to my family because I wouldn't get any from him.

I was terrified about what was happening to me. Was I going to be a giant? Would the surgery kill me? Would the destruction of my pituitary and its hormonal consequences change my personality? Would I be able to care for my children? Would I be able to carry on working? My consultant didn't know the answers to these questions.

I needed comfort and reassurance from my husband that he would be with me through this ordeal; unfortunately that was not on the menu in our marriage. So my attitude to him changed. He had grown up in South Africa and was accustomed to servants and subservient women. Only eight days after my son was born, I asked him to carry the dustbin out to the collection point at the front of the house. He refused to do it, and so I had to struggle to do it myself. After my son was born, though, things began to change. I was maturing fast and becoming extremely independent. I became more assertive, and this offended his sensibilities. With his superior sense of self-value, he was very put off when he had to iron his own shirts or when he would drop his underwear on the bathroom floor and I did not tidy up after him. I decided enough was enough. I waited until there were five or six pairs of dirty knickers in the bathroom, scooped them up and put them in his briefcase after he'd packed his sandwiches. At lunch time they all fell out onto the office floor. Needless to say, he was not pleased. Surprisingly he started to put his dirty washing in the laundry basket. While I survived my illness, the marriage didn't. He spent more and more time seeking younger, prettier partners in good health – something that had probably always been in plain view had I but seen it.

I met my present husband in 1994. He loved me for myself – and still does.

Life as a Mom

Both my pregnancies were horrible. I felt like I wanted to crawl into a corner and not come out again until it was all over. It felt like I was chronically depressed and had no energy. Some mothers have postpartum depression due to confused hormones, but mine was definitely pre-natal. My hormones obviously worked well enough to support the babies: both good birth weights and healthy.

After both births, I produced milk in vast quantities – so much so that any extra amount was sent off to the local special care baby unit. I stopped feeding my second child when he was eight months old, but I carried on producing colostrum continually until he was twelve. Blood tests revealed my prolactin levels were "normal." Not normal for me obviously, but of no concern to the medical professionals.

When I was a young mom, I had lots of energy. Besides raising my own two children, I was a nanny for another four children. It was great fun. Come rain or shine, we would make daily trips to the park or, in the summer, frequent train rides to the seaside. Wherever I went, I was constantly counting heads to ensure nobody was lagging behind or lost. I'd have two little ones in the buggy, a toddler hanging on each side, and two old enough to run on ahead. I'd have swim suits, towels, and a huge picnic to carry too. Happy days! When the children started school, I was doing the school run, on foot, four times a day. I was exceptionally fit and very slim though I was still having headaches, aching legs and just didn't feel 'well'.

Medical Problems for My Child

My daughter was diagnosed with Still's Disease (Systemic-Onset Juvenile Rheumatoid Arthritis) when she was only three years old. She couldn't walk due to the swelling in her right knee. She frequently complained of pain in her right jaw and elbow although there was no visible swelling in these joints. The orthopedic consultant told me that she could become blind, crippled, and in permanent need of a wheelchair. If she got really bad, she would need to be on prescribed steroids that would make her fat and cause her hair to fall out. The doctor did give us hope though. He said that it was possible for her to grow out of it by the time she was 13. While any damage done would be permanent, the idea of her growing out of it was still where we held our hope.

At the doctor's advice, I gave her aspirin three times a day to curb the inflammation. I was worried that she would get a stomach ulcer from this dosage, but I was told that it was necessary, and that they would just deal with the ulcer when it happened. The doctor said at the end of the appointment that I should take her home and keep her in bed for three weeks. I was so angry that as a mother I should be expected to manage such a grim prognosis for my daughter! Luckily, I guess, I was not diagnosed with Acromegaly yet, so I didn't have to manage the psychology of both of our illnesses at the same time. I knew that I had to manage my attitude though. Forever the proactive optimist, I bought her a pair of roller skates on the way home! After much thought about what I could do, I took her to see a Homeopath. He told me that he could guarantee a cure for eczema, asthma and osteoarthritis, but was not so sure about Still's Disease. His advice was to put her on a "cleansing" diet – I suppose what passes for "detox" nowadays – for two weeks. She also had these tiny little pills to take daily – I don't know what they were – but such a small pill that I had to pick them up with tweezers. I had always cooked proper food for my children, so she was used to eating lots of fruit, salad, and vegetables. She was only three. I explained to her about the diet, and what it would do. I'm sure, even at that young age, she understood and readily agreed to the new regiment.

After the "cleansing" all her symptoms had gone. No swelling. No pain. The Homeopath suggested I keep her on a vegetarian, whole food diet. I figured that if nothing else, it would keep her healthy and help her body cope with the disease. I kept up the hospital appointments with orthopedic consultant who could see the results of what I was doing, but evidence of the disease was in every blood test until she was eight.

She was seven when I was diagnosed with Acromegaly. I was not totally honest with her about my condition, but despite my reassurances, she was convinced I was going to die, and she suffered months of night terrors—and it was only me who got up to comfort her, shaking, tearful, and trapped in her nightmares. Her father had no concern for her mental health or my lack of sleep. It was a very trying time for me and my daughter. I was dealing with her fear, my fear—and his rejection of both of us. My son was too young to grasp what was happening, but he was brave in his own right, scaring away burglars, breaking into the kitchen in the middle of the night right around the same time as all our medical struggles.

As I struggled to manage my children, their health, my marriage and its health, my self-esteem took a nose dive and it was only a successful business career that restored me.

Relationships with My Childhood Family as an Adult

Relationships with my father and step-mother had improved considerably after I left home, as they no longer had any power in my life. It would be wrong and unfair if I did not say that I am very grateful for the help and support they gave to me and my children throughout my illness.

After all the force-feeding of religion and the blatant hypocrisy that surrounded me as a child, I rebelled against the Lord and was atheist for many years. Now, though, I cannot continue this story without thanking God for His loving kindness; even when I rejected him, He loved and cared for me.

Today

Menstruation was and still is a very real problem for me. Heavy bleeding, irregularity and severe pain are normal features of my period. When I was 34 I was given a drug to counter this, but it actually stopped menstruation completely. It wasn't supposed to do this, but I was delighted to have the break from my periods since they had always made my life more unbearable than it already was. Under supervision from the hospital, I kept taking the same drug for eight years regardless of the fact that the recommended usage period is three months, and this drug was known to cause blood clots. In spite of this, I took it continually until I had a stroke in 1997. No one wanted to confirm that the prolonged taking of the drug caused it, but I am convinced that it was the cause. After I stopped taking the drug, menstruation returned with a vengeance—worse than before; heavier bleeding, more pain, and still very irregular.

I have been to see two gynecologists where I live now, in Dorset. Neither of them had heard of Acromegaly, and the absence of a pituitary gland baffled them both completely. One even suggested Hormone Replacement Therapy – just what I didn't want when I have menopause *and excess hormones* from Acromegaly. I think that at this point I have given up. What I need is a gynecological endocrinologist – and since they do not have any kind of endocrinologist in my county, there is little chance of that happening for me.

I now see an endocrinologist every year. Six weeks before my appointment I have a test to check cortisol levels in my body. This test is an injection into muscle to provoke the adrenal glands into action—producing raised blood levels of cortisol. It's really like fright by injection! In 2007 the laboratory that analyzes the blood samples – one taken before injection and one taken thirty minutes after – sent an incomplete set of results to the consultant. They had sent the "before" results, showing normal levels of cortisol. Unfortunately and, I suppose, logically, the consultant assumed they were the "after" results and gave me a letter for my doctor requesting that I be prescribed steroid tablets and a supply of syringes and vials of adrenalin in case of collapse. Meanwhile, my doctor had a complete set of results but decided to go along with what the consultant had requested, even though he did not consider the steroids necessary. A letter was sent to the consultant with the complete results. The wheels of the National Health System move very slowly, and it was about three months before I received a letter telling me to wean myself off the steroids very slowly. In the meantime, my husband was too worried about me to leave me on my own and put his life on hold to ensure I hung on to mine.

It turned out that I didn't need the steroids. The effects were ghastly. I had acne on my face, neck and back. Hair sprouted in all the places a lady doesn't want it. I suffered panic attacks and palpitations. I put on weight, which was a real bummer since I had just managed to lose forty-two pounds. I was also very depressed. I felt like I'd taken a big slide down the slope to decrepitude. I knew that, despite everything I saw on the outside, there was still a pretty, slim, dainty, five foot six inch female inside me, and I was pretty sure that I hadn't eaten her! It is how I see myself in my head, and despite constant reminders from mirrors and other people, it is still my mental image of myself. I am sure it is not my deliberate delusion, but my brain is reacting to what happened to my body and refusing to change the template. When I go clothes shopping now, I always make sure I take a tape measure because I have been known to purchase clothes that were too small just because they really did look like they would fit.

I have often been mistaken for a man because of my height and build, and I would like to say I am used to it, but it still hurts. I have very broad shoulders. I love it when padded shoulders are in fashion. I take them out and the garment is a really good fit. I tend to stay away from mirrors and photographers. The facial changes caused by Acromegaly are amplified in photographs, making me look like a cartoon ogre!

I was exceptionally strong for a female. I worked for an office equipment supplier and could easily lift and carry boxes of A3 size paper, as well as help the guys shift the photocopying machines. My strength lasted a long time. When my son was a teenager of considerable build he challenged me to arm wrestle him in front of his mates. Much to his chagrin and his friends' amusement. I won. I bought him a set of weights as a consolation prize!

The worst thing about Acromegaly, for me, is the lack of available information. When I was first diagnosed, the medical world was only expecting males to get it. Even after I was diagnosed, it was like my doctors were learning about Acromegaly alongside me. Nowadays, things are easier because there is the internet and online groups where sufferers can talk to one another worldwide. The benefit for me has been huge.

Living My Life while Managing My Disease

I don't know whether the medical professionals didn't know or didn't tell me, but I was never informed that my cartilage would be unable to take the weight of my bones. A recent x-ray of my spine and neck showed degenerative disc disease and arthritis. My knees, elbows and right hip are on the way out. This deficiency affects the way I live considerably. I have arthritis in my neck and jaw. Every cough or sneeze causes extreme pain. I am unable to yawn properly and can't open my mouth that wide without aggravating the arthritic inflammation. I have swallowing difficulty because of the stroke, and everything I eat much be chewed to a pulp before I attempt to swallow, so sometimes I have to live on soup alone. Even everyday tasks like showering and dressing are difficult and painful. I need help with putting on lower body garments, since I can't bend my spine sufficiently to reach down far enough for pants and socks.

To help me, I have a litter-picker (sometimes known as long-reach) so I can reach to remove garments more easily, but I still can't untie bootlaces or remove boots from my feet. I have a special frame around the lavatory so I can sit down and get up without assistance. I am unable to help carry the groceries or put the rubbish out. I never attempt to lift anything heavier than my cat. I get really frustrated at times, having to rely on someone else's good nature to help me to carry out what others consider everyday normal functions. I need to do the laundry, my husband has to deliver the laundry to the machine. I have an office chair with wheels in my kitchen. The chair is set to its lowest height so I can reach into the washing machine, oven and cupboards without having to bend. The work surfaces in the kitchen are raised to accommodate my height. The sofas in my lounge are on blocks so I don't have too far to sit down or overuse my knees to stand up from a sitting position.

There are rails on both sides of the stairs so I can use my arms to take some of the weight off of my knees and allegedly, to stop my lazy stroke foot from tripping me up. I have scoliosis due to an injury caused by weak lefthand side muscles after the stroke. I was told to expect diabetes and the loss of all my teeth by the time I was forty, but I do not have diabetes and still have most of my teeth.

My weight is a continual problem. It's bad enough having to hunt for long-leg trousers – I don't want to be fat as well. I gain body mass without overeating—I seem to have the same metabolic rate as a hibernating sloth! I am unable to exercise much because of chronic back pain and the wear and tear caused to all my joints. When I take a short walk, I have to lay down for a couple of hours to recuperate. I can't sit in the car for more than 45 minutes without my vertebrae locking.

My eyes are still extremely light sensitive. The only bit of me that has shrunk significantly is my jaw. I still feel big and ugly although my dear husband assures me I'm not. He's either just being kind or needs new spectacles. My teeth are now next to each other. I have a very thick skull with corners on it!

Luckily, my Acromegaly is cured. The only relevant medication I still take is thyroxine. My biggest worries are the lack of menopause, increasingly limited mobility and the half-life of the radiation that destroyed the tumour working its magic on the surrounding areas of brain tissue. Apparently the radiation is effective for about twenty years and the poisonous effect it had on the tumour lives on.

My Virtual Friends, and Real Peace of Mind

I have never met anyone else who has had Acromegaly. I had always felt totally isolated until I discovered the internet support group on Facebook. I believe I am the oldest person in the group and as such have been able to encourage others who have only recently been diagnosed.

Having Acromegaly is like jumping out of an airplane without a parachute: a real leap into the unknown. I am glad I have been able via Facebook to use my experiences to offer support to others. I am sure changes in appearance affect men and women to the same degree, but we girls are supposed to make the most of ourselves whereas it is okay for men to go around looking like Fungus the Bogeyman! A man having a big square jaw might be hereditary and still look normal, but for us girls, it can destroy our image of our femininity.

I believe the best way to deal with Acromegaly and its tidal wave of after-effects is to look upon oneself as a survivor, not a victim. Stay positive.

Jaki Loebig is retired after a successful career in computing and management, due to a stroke. Born in London, England, she now lives happily, with her loving husband, in a picturesque village on the Dorset coast. As a veteran survivor of Acromegaly she is struggling, and mostly winning, with the after effects of the illness, i.e., degenerative cartilage disease and arthritis.

Career Issues

Ellen K.

I don't like work—no man does—but I like what is in the work—the chance to find yourself. Your own reality—for yourself not for others—what no other man can ever know. They can only see the mere show, and never can tell what it really means.

—Joseph Conrad (Heart of Darkness)

Hello! My name is Ellen, and I go by "POLARCHIP" on the Internet. I started my blog, polarchip.blogspot.com, in July of 2005 with no particular intention, and then later that same month I was diagnosed with Acromegaly. I have been documenting my life and my experience with the Acromegaly ever since. The diagnosis was a complete shock, as I had been concerned about almost every classic symptom of Acromegaly for a while, but my doctor had dismissed each symptom individually, most of them attributed to stress. When I finally did get a proper diagnosis, I was terrified by the unknown and rareness of the disease. Through the "blogosphere," I started meeting others who have been affected, and in January of 2007, I created acromegalybloggers.blogspot.com to raise awareness of the disease and to provide information and support to those who have been affected by it.

I wanted to write this chapter because my Acromegaly and my career have been deeply intertwined. My Acromegaly has impacted my career in numerous ways, and my career has impacted my Acromegaly. I struggle with both, and I hope that by sharing what

I have learned in the process, I can help make other people's lives a little easier.

About two weeks before I found out I had Acromegaly, I went into my manager's office to quit my job. I was twenty-six years old at the time, and I sat in front of my manager in tears because I was totally fed up. I constantly felt drained and had headaches, which I thought were a result of dealing with so much on-the-job stress. My feet were swollen and had grown a full size and width—I thought it was because at work I was on my feet for hours and hours at a time. I had joint pain in my neck and shoulders that I thought was from hunching over a computer all the time. In general I felt terrible. I'm incredibly fortunate that my manager liked me, because instead of accepting my two-week notice, he suggested I take two weeks of unpaid leave to think it over and reconsider staying. I had nothing to lose, so I accepted his offer.

When I think about that moment now, I realize that it was a point where my life took a huge turn and that the outcome of my life could have been dramatically different.

If I hadn't had those two extra weeks of health insurance and free time, my diagnosis could have taken several more years, or I could have discovered that I had Acromegaly when I had no health coverage. In a way, because my manager offered me those two extra weeks, I avoided potential disaster. I was intending to drop all my health insurance when I quit, figuring that I was relatively young and that all of my health complaints were a result of my job. I figured I should get a new pair of glasses before I left, though, because I had been noticing that my vision had become blurry. I scheduled an exam with an optometrist, but when my new glasses arrived, I was disappointed that the new prescription didn't seem to help the blurriness problem at all.

I thought that perhaps seasonal allergies were causing the blurriness, or in the worst case that I had some kind of scratch on my cornea, so I decided to go to an ophthalmologist to look into the issue further, figuring I would walk out with a prescription for special eye drops or something like that. The ophthalmologist who examined me was a very young doctor who seemed new to the office. When she examined my eyes, she seemed perplexed by the fact that even with the right glasses, my vision wasn't normal. I was seeing about 20/30, and I remember her saying, "There's no reason why someone your age shouldn't be able to see 20/20 with correction." This was another moment when the outcome of my life could have easily taken a different course; if the ophthalmologist had not been diligent about investigating my impairment of vision, the Acromegaly could have gone undetected for several more years. She ordered several additional tests which were performed right away.

I looked into machines that shined lights into my eyes while the doctor looked at the surface and the back of each eye. She couldn't find anything abnormal there, so I took a vision test that seemed to be almost like a video game—I clicked a button every time I saw a flashing light inside a dimly lit cave. I found out later that this "game" was called a Humphrey visual field test. I had no idea what this test was looking for, but when the doctor was reviewing the results, she became quiet and concerned. She showed me the resulting graph with big black blotches in the outer quadrant of each eye's field of vision where I had missed every flashing light. She explained that this pattern of vision loss indicated that my optic nerve was being compressed. I found the idea to be completely absurd. I jokingly asked her what could possibly be pressing on my optic nerve, "a tumor?!" I expected her to laugh and assure me that it couldn't possibly be something like that. But she just looked back at me very seriously and said that it was a possibility, and I would need more tests to find out. I left the office that day with a referral to see a neuro-ophthalmologist at the local university hospital. When I met with the doctor, he reviewed my previous vision tests, looked in my eyes, and waved his fingers in front of me while I looked at his nose. Finally he ordered an MRI and blood work. When the results came back, they found a pituitary tumor and elevated growth hormone levels. I was diagnosed with Acromegaly and scheduled for the next available surgery date.

I went back to see my manager at the end of my two-week unpaid leave and explained my diagnosis. Instead of quitting I was able to take a medical leave of absence so that I could undergo surgery and recover while remaining insured. Everyone at work was shocked by the news of what had happened, but they were all incredibly supportive and kind. I still look back in amazement when I think about what would have happened to me if I had discovered the Acromegaly after I had quit and had no health insurance. I don't know if my manager truly appreciates how the offer of the two-week leave forever changed my life, but I am eternally grateful.

Waiting for surgery was probably the hardest period of my Acromegaly journey. Before my pituitary surgery, I had never been in the hospital for anything more severe than a mole removal, so having surgery in such a vulnerable area of the body—deep inside the head—seemed so dangerous. All of a sudden I felt like my surgery day was a very clearly defined date when I might die, and it was up to me to make peace with the world in those few weeks. Knowing what I now know about how advanced the techniques are, I realize how relatively safe the surgery is, and I wouldn't hesitate to have the surgery again if I thought I could be fully cured. But at the time, I was filled with fear of the unknown and even had a full anxiety attack a week before my surgery. I had an extreme splitting headache that landed me in the emergency room because doctors were afraid that it might be the tumor hemorrhaging. In hindsight, this was probably the one time where stress really was the culprit of a headache. I spent the night under observation, and from then on I had no hesitation taking the anti-anxiety tablets that my GP had prescribed for me back when I first broke into tears explaining how my eye exam had led to my Acromegaly diagnosis. I had expressed my fear of the surgery, and the anti-anxiety pills were prescribed as something to have on hand if needed. I had been reluctant to take them before, but obviously they helped a lot when I was completely freaking out; and even before I took them, it was comforting to know I had them available.

If waiting for surgery was the hardest part of my Acromegaly journey, then the easiest part was actually having the surgery. I don't remember a thing from the surgery, and all the hard work was in the hands of my surgeons. I drifted off to sleep looking up at my anesthesiologist, who was patting my cheek. I assume he was smiling at me because the corners of his eyes crinkled when I looked at him (the surgical mask covered the rest of his face). After that, I woke up in the ICU under observation. Recovery was tough, as I had a potassium deficiency, which meant I needed a potassium IV, which was extremely painful. I could feel the liquid burning in my veins. Other than the potassium, there were no complications such as a CSF leak, diabetes insipidus, or infection. After a day or two, I went to a regular hospital room. Before the surgery, I imagined recovery would mean I would be sitting up in bed, receiving a line of visitors waiting to give me flowers and hugs. In reality, I didn't want to see or talk to anyone because I was such a mess. I'm relieved that very few people saw me in that state. The few people who did see me (all family) never revealed how miserable I looked. I didn't look in a mirror until my last day in the hospital, and I was shocked by my appearance—my nose and cheeks had swollen to cartoonish dimensions. After another few days, I still couldn't quite walk confidently, but the hospital discharged me anyway because I was medically stable. After I went home, my boyfriend (now husband!) took care of me until I had my strength back.

After I fully recovered from surgery, I still wasn't sure I could go back to "work as usual." I felt uncomfortable going back because I still held a lot of emotional baggage from that workplace. I had developed deep anxiety issues, and I felt like a needed a fresh start, but I didn't know what to do next. I was living in New York at the time, and my manager helped me obtain a transfer performing the same role, but two thousand miles away in California.

I packed up my things and started out on what I thought was my new life in Los Angeles. I thought I had overcome my brush with mortality, and none of my new friends (mostly co-workers) knew about my tumor or my surgery, and so it was easy to pretend that none of it had ever happened. I found happiness in my new environment, but several months later my Acromegaly caught up with me all the way across the country when my neurosurgeon's office called to tell me that my latest MRI showed that I had residual tumor present and my growth hormone levels were still high.

The shock of being told that I still had residual tumor after the surgeon had previously described the operation as "beautiful" and "perfect" came out of the blue. I thought the surgery was completely successful at removing the entire tumor, so the news was completely devastating. I thought making it through surgery meant that I had dodged a bullet, but hearing that I had residual tumor was almost like I was being diagnosed all over again. My father, who had accompanied me to the pre-operation consultation with my surgeon, reminded me that the doctor had mentioned there was only a thirty percent chance that the surgery would be completely successful, but there were so many other thoughts swirling through my mind, I had no recollection of that comment. I'm glad I had someone with me for that consultation who was slightly more detached from the situation and could help me remember those details later.

I was told that I needed radiation, but since I was living alone in a completely new city, I didn't think I would be able to handle driving myself to treatments and being so far away from family and friends. I took another medical leave of absence so I could go back to New York (where I had been living when I was diagnosed) and pursued radiation there. Just like when I was faced with surgery, fear of the unknown plagued my mind. Would my optic nerve be damaged? Would I lose all my hair? Would I have burns from the radiation? Would the radiation be successful? Would the radiation cause secondary tumors? I felt all my old anxiety welling up inside me again.

When I told my new manager, he was completely shocked because as far as he knew, I was completely healthy. It was hard to explain the severity of the disease, and even though he was probably one of the best managers I have ever worked for, he seemed uncomfortable when I talked about my condition. I don't know if there were legal liabilities for the company if I talked to him about it or if he was just scared or overwhelmed to think about tumors (it can make people uncomfortable). Even though he didn't seem too eager to know more, he was very supportive and helped me get my medical leave sorted out.

I went for my radiation consultations in New York, but at the last minute, my doctors decided that I should postpone radiation and pursue medication treatment first, so I agreed and returned to work. Even though I loved the manager and the work environment that I returned to, I ended up requesting another transfer. My boyfriend and I were having a long-distance relationship between Los Angeles and the San Francisco Bay Area, but after the episode considering radiation, I wanted to be closer to loved ones. Since I had a great performance record, getting another transfer was easy. I had met lots of great friends through the job in L.A., and even though they were sad I was leaving, everyone understood why I needed to move.

My enthusiasm for my job went quickly downhill at the new location. The manager there was mostly incompetent, or maybe it was just disappointment, having come from such a great environment just previously. In addition, going through my medical drama made me realize that I couldn't handle the physical demands of that job (standing for long hours, lifting, climbing ladders, dealing with the public, etc.) on a long term basis, and I knew I needed to move on to a different kind of job. I began getting really stressed out—which never helps with health situations—because I was terrified of quitting. The last time I had tried to quit, I found out I had a brain tumor, so there were some pretty deep negative associations there. On the other hand, I also became afraid of being fired one day if I wasn't able to keep up with the fast pace of the business.

I continued to stress about health insurance coverage because I didn't fully understand what *COBRA*, *preexisting condition*, *period of creditable coverage*, or any of the other insurance jargon meant. I just knew that if anything happened to my health insurance, I would go bankrupt trying to pay for my medications, tests, and doctors' appointments out-of-pocket. Taking another step towards the unknown was something that I tried to avoid at all costs, and I became simultaneously miserable at work but paralyzed by fear of moving on. There are lots of laws and resources in place to protect employees from losing health coverage, and as I took the time to understand what all these terms meant, it helped take the pressure off of feeling like I was trapped.

Through the support of my loved ones, I was eventually able to take the leap to a new job. The new job was a vast improvement because there was much less physical activity (it was more of a desk job). But the commute was horrible, and trying to schedule tests or appointments with my doctor was difficult because I was already losing so many hours in the day just to the commute. At this point, I was a little more confident about switching jobs since I had done it once successfully, and I had also learned a little more about how the health insurance system works; so I left for a new job.

I have switched jobs a few more times since then, and today I work for one of the best employers in the world. I get great health benefits, have a lot of flexibility in my schedule, and my manager is supportive, kind, understanding, and aware of my Acromegaly (although I don't know how deep her understanding of the disease is). Even though I have come an incredibly long way, the work I do is occasionally high-stress, emotionally draining, and physically demanding—much like at the job I held when I was first diagnosed. Sometimes I still worry about the effect of stress on my overall health since my growth hormone levels are still not fully controlled despite surgery and increasing doses of medication. I'm not sure what my next options are, but I am working with my doctor, and I am also looking into "alternative" therapies. I have considered taking time off from work so that I can focus on my health full time, but for now I am able to keep working.

So in general things are pretty good, but I'm still asking myself where I want to go with my career; and balancing work with life, health, and family is still a struggle. Let's be clear. For me, working is not a choice; it is a necessity. Obvious considerations like income aside, health insurance is a huge factor despite changes to the US health care system in March 2010. I have found some unexpected side benefits to staying active in the workforce despite having Acromegaly, and even if income and health insurance weren't an issue, I like to think I would still keep working.

It's really easy to feel disadvantaged in a competitive workplace because people with Acromegaly have so much more to deal with than most people. Often times having Acromegaly feels like a job in itself because of the fatigue; the side effects of medication; the symptoms; and the time spent going to doctors, having tests, filling prescriptions, and dealing with the other extra care that is required. I could go on and on, but I imagine that most people reading this are already too aware of the challenges that Acromegaly presents. I've made a point to try and find the upside of the challenges of working while dealing with Acromegaly, and I'll share my thoughts here.

Challenges might mean that I have to work harder, but they have also helped me discover who I really am. I realize how precious life is now, and it's made me really reevaluate why I do the work I do. I have become very selective about the way I spend my time; for example, being with loved ones is much more valuable to me than spending an extra hour in my office, trying to inch ahead in the company. I've learned to appreciate everyday life, and I seek work that is meaningful to me. One of the drawbacks to performing work you're really passionate about is that there is an inherent level of stress that comes along with it, because you care so much; but if I'm not passionate about something, it's really hard for me to stay motivated when energy is already hard to come by.

Sometimes just getting out of bed is really hard for me, and if I had no one to be accountable to, I might just stay in bed all day. As tempting as it sounds, I know that actually staying in bed all day isn't good for me or anyone else. Knowing that I need to be somewhere at a specific time gives me the little push I need to face the world. This is a great example of a challenge that work presents but that ultimately makes my life better.

Being in bed all day would also mean being home alone all day, and I know that being alone for so long can spiral into isolation and depression. In my opinion, depression is one of the most unacknowledged symptoms of Acromegaly. I like seeing and interacting with my co-workers, and since most of the people I work with have no idea that I have any kind of medical issue, they treat me as they would any other co-worker. They don't look at me with worrying concern, and they don't walk on eggshells when talking about health-related subjects, so I feel like I get uncensored honesty from them. When I'm feeling good, I can simply focus on my responsibilities and feel "normal."

In that way, work provides a great distraction from my health issues, and it can help keep me from wallowing in self-pity. Sometimes, we need to have something to focus on other than ourselves and Acromegaly, and work can provide that.

My career is still a work in progress, and ultimately, deciding where to go with any career is a deeply personal process. Sometimes I feel like I may not be able to work because of Acromegaly, and sometimes I feel like I can't stop working because of Acromegaly. It is possible to manage having both a career and Acromegaly, but throughout it all, it has been vital that HEALTH COMES FIRST because if you don't place health first, everything else (including your work) suffers.

....

Additional Random Thoughts on Acromegaly and the Workplace

Stress

I believe that stress is as toxic for the body as environmental toxins, so I try really hard to keep perspective on what is worth stressing over and what is not. I suspect that hormone imbalance contributes to stress, and stress contributes to hormone imbalance, which can create a dangerous feedback loop, so it's really important to take control of your emotional well being.

It's impossible to avoid stress completely, so we have to confront it head-on. Everyone deals with stress differently, and there are some approaches that are healthier than others. If you can, try to take breaks, stretch, go outside for fresh air and a walk, or talk to a friend. Regular exercise also helps, as does meditation/prayer. If your job is inherently stressful, maybe you should consider finding a new job.

Having a career can mean added stress from office pressures, responsibilities, and deadlines. Most of my perfectly healthy friends complain about how stressful their jobs are and how hard it is to balance work and life, so I know this isn't unique to people with Acromegaly. Having a major medical issue to deal with on top of everything can mean two things: either it can contribute to your stress, or it can make you realize that all the things that people get upset about at work are trivial. In the big picture, most of our office drama is inconsequential compared to ensuring your own health.

That doesn't mean all the stress from work magically disappeared once I realized this. I have taken stress management classes and gone to individual counseling, and both have significantly improved my quality of life. In a lot of ways, being diagnosed with Acromegaly was traumatic for me, and I felt that I had a lot of issues similar to those diagnosed with posttraumatic stress disorder (PTSD). Taking an active effort to control my emotions and finding strategies to deal with stress have really helped me feel like the "real me" again, from before I was diagnosed.

Symptoms

There are so many symptoms of Acromegaly that have a direct impact on productivity. For me, I struggle with fatigue and depression, which I sometimes confuse with lack of motivation or lack of ambition. At my first job, I attributed my headaches, neck pain, and foot growth to workplace conditions, but they were really due to Acromegaly. The same can happen elsewhere. If I'm not feeling well, I ask myself, is this the Acromegaly or is this the job? Some of my work pains that are also side effects of Acromegaly are carpal tunnel syndrome and neck and shoulder stiffness. It is my responsibility to make sure I am careful of work circumstances that may be detrimental to my health, such as lifting heavy objects, standing for long periods of time, and repetitive stress.

Managing Work and Medical Demands

Calling to schedule appointments, getting lab results, ordering prescriptions, or disputing insurance billing issues takes time, and a lot of offices and services are only open during business hours. This means that work time and time for taking care of your health have to overlap! Calling medical offices can be awkward if you sit in an open cubicle with your officemates, so if you don't have one already, I suggest getting a cell phone and only using that number when filling out contact information with your healthcare providers.

Privacy

Before I told my current manager about my Acromegaly, I wrestled with the decision to bring it up or not. On one hand, I didn't want to be treated differently than my colleagues. For example, I didn't want my capabilities to be put into question, which might mean I would miss opportunities because people would be concerned that I wouldn't be able to handle them. I worried that my manager, though well intentioned, would treat me with kid gloves or worry about me. On the other hand, there have been times when I needed to take time away from the office to attend to my health; and my performance has sometimes suffered because I was simply in pain, overcome with fatigue, or having side effects from medication; thus, I needed special consideration. I wonder how this has affected my opportunities for moving ahead.

Sometimes I wish I could tell people at work so that when I take time off for my appointments, they know it's for something serious and that I'm not just slacking off. Also, sometimes I really feel terrible (headaches, fatigue, joint pain) and I wish I could tell them so they don't think I'm just being lazy or sullen.

Many of the symptoms of Acromegaly are invisible to others. The headaches, joint aches, pains, fatigue, depression, and vision defects do not affect outward appearance, but they do affect quality of work, the ability to work longer hours, and motivation.

For the observable symptoms such as enlarged feet, hands, jaw, acne, sweat, odor, or extreme height (for those with gigantism), coworkers may notice not realize that they are a result of a serious medical condition or they may suspect it but feel uncomfortable bringing it up. Appearances are important in the workplace (there have been studies about attractiveness and success in job interviews or promotions), so I wonder if there is discrimination when visible body changes occur.

Solutions to Challenges

Right Job

I mentioned how Acromegaly has forced me to step back from my life and reassess what is important to me. When I think about how Acromegaly may shorten my life, … I now perform work that I know helps people and changes lives for the better, and it's very gratifying to get feedback from the people that I help. I'm not sure I could stay motivated doing something that I consider trivial, just to earn a paycheck.

One "job" that I have taken on since I've been diagnosed with Acromegaly is becoming an advocate for Acromegaly patients. When I think about performing work that I consider important, I can think of nothing more important than helping others who have been in the same situation as me, and I am passionate about finding a cure for Acromegaly. I don't have medical or chemistry training, so I do what I can do—spread the word and raise awareness.

Good Manager

I've heard the saying, "You don't quit your job, you quit your manager," and I think there's a lot of truth behind it. A lot of times my ability to enjoy the work I do depends on the direction, support, and acknowledgment that I get from my direct manager. I have had several managers since I was diagnosed, and I have informed some of them about my Acromegaly, and some of them still have no idea. Some of my managers have been fantastic, and some have been nightmares to work for, but the ones who were fantastic were not necessarily the ones that I told, and the ones that were nightmares were not necessarily the ones I didn't tell.

One of the great managers that I worked for gave me a lot of freedom to take care of business on my own, and he knew that I was responsible enough to take care of business no matter what, so there was never a need to tell them about my Acromegaly- He simply trusted me to take care of business.

Of the managers I have told, it's been difficult to explain to them how serious Acromegaly is. I never know how in depth to go when describing what causes it, what the symptoms are. Usually their eyes glaze over once I get to *pituitary tumor*. Some of my mangers have not been allowed to discuss my medical situation at length because of company concerns about potential discrimination. In those cases, there has always been someone from Human Resources that I could talk to confidentially. It's good to just let someone be aware of the situation so that if issues come up later on, you have it on record that someone at the company was aware.

I think this advice goes out to anyone who is in the workplace regardless of health issues- make sure you feel like your manager has your best interests in mind. If you aren't getting what you need from your manager, talk to someone higher up, look into a transfer, or consider switching companies.

- No matter how great your manager is, sometimes your manager's support can be limited by company policies and resources. For most of my career, I have worked for large technology companies so I've been fortunate to have progressive attitudes in my workplace and good benefits. Some examples of benefits I get beyond the standard health insurance are onsite physical therapy and ergonomic evaluations (having my desk, monitor, and chair adjusted has improved my neck and shoulder pain).
- The company culture also dictates attitudes towards work/life balance, so keep that in mind if you are considering companies to work for.
- I think working for a larger, more established company makes it easier to deal with health issues because there is more structure and precedent for dealing with it. On the other hand, if you work for a smaller or newer company, it may be difficult for your company to figure out what to do when faced with special requests, but it could also mean that you may have more freedom and options.
- If your company does not value you, you should consider moving on. It may be tough to look for new work, but it's definitely worth it in the long run.
- In addition to the benefits, make sure you have a good contact in HR that helps keep you informed of what benefits are available, how to handle tough situations where you don't feel comfortable talking to your manager or anyone else on your team, and if the time comes, discussions about long or short term disability leave.

Flexible Schedule

I feel incredibly fortunate that I am able to maintain a flexible schedule that allows me to attend my appointments with my doctors, have tests done, pick up prescriptions, and whatever else I need to do to stay on top of my health. This means I end up working on the weekends or in the evenings from time to time, but I appreciate that I don't have to adhere to arbitrary business hours.

Telecommuting is another way to gain flexibility in your schedule. When you don't have to physically be in an office, you can work in a more comfortable environment, which can also help with repetitive stress injuries (carpal tunnel is a symptom of Acromegaly), sore joints, etc. I find I can work more comfortably and longer hours when I sit with my computer in bed.

Right now, traveling for work is difficult for me, because if I'm away during the week when I'm supposed to get my shot, I either have to take the shot a few days early or a few days late. My doctor says that it's no big deal to shift a few days either way, but I feel the effects - either the side effects of the medication emerge or I feel Acromegaly symptoms. I prefer to take my medication exactly on schedule (I take the shot every three weeks, usually on a Wednesday), which means it's hard to fit work travel around my shot. I plan to avoid business travel in any future jobs. I know that I could potentially take the shot with me, but keeping it refrigerated and then finding a nurse in to administer the shot in whatever town I'm seems like a huge hassle. I enjoy traveling, but Acromegaly has definitely put restrictions on my sense of freedom. I know that drug companies are working on better solutions, so right now I am keeping my hopes up that something better will come out soon.

Having a good commute is another way to make the work day a little easier on yourself- for a while I spent 1.5 hours every morning and every evening on the CalTrain (Northern California commuter rail) to get to my job, which was almost as physically draining as the job I had left because of the physical demands! Adding 3 hours to my 9 hour work day meant that I left home and returned home in the dark during the winter months, and I would have to take the entire day off if I had a doctor's appointment, because it was not worth it to do a 3 hour commute just to work a half day.

Helpful Tools and Resources

I have found that keeping an online calendar has been helpful for me to keep track of my work demands and my medical appointments, blood draws, and medication times. I have three separate online calendars, one for work, one for personal, and one dedicated solely to health, and I can overlay them to see in advance when any potential conflicts might come up.

My medical provider has great online tools for scheduling, viewing, and canceling appointments, along with email reminders. They also let you refill prescriptions online and check the status of each one. Since it is a HMO, I don't have to worry about billing between the health insurance and the doctor, pharmacy, or laboratory, and I know that pretty much everything is covered as long as I stay in network. For those who have to deal with billing, I have heard of services like health care concierges or case managers that take of all that for you. I know first hand how frustrating it can be to be the go-between when there are billing/approval issues among the insurance, doctor, pharmacy, laboratory, and hospital.

The HR department at my company has also been very helpful in working with me and my doctor to accommodate my health care concerns and needs. They can help with medical leaves, work modifications, work accommodations, or even transfers to new roles. I was recently granted a work accommodation from my company, which was a huge relief for me because it means that there are specific limitations to what I can be expected to do (overtime is no longer expected, I can have compensation time for time spent traveling, etc). This has been useful for helping me maintain work/life balance. It took a bit of work and back and forth between my doctor and the HR department, but in the end it was worth it. I haven't had to make any drastic changes yet, but it acts as a safety net for me, and knowing it is there relieves a lot of the stress I have associated with dealing with a chronic medical issue.

Family, friends, doctors, nurses, and others in the Acromegaly community are also there for you, but you should not depend on them to take care of everything. I have an incredible husband who reminds me when I'm due for my shot and helps me with my injections, which is great, but I can't expect him to revolve his whole life around my Acromegaly. Remember that even though you have people around to help, ultimately YOU are the one who is most responsible for your own health, so rely on others but don't depend on them! Take charge and be a proactive champion for your own well being.

I hope for all of us that there will be a complete and permanent cure for Acromegaly and one day the disease will no longer exist. Till then, live your life to the fullest possible and good luck!

Ellen was diagnosed with Acromegaly in 2005 and has been an active advocate in the community ever since. Her acromegalybloggers.blogspot.com has been an invaluable resource for patients around the world, both to read and to post their thoughts, feelings, and occasional frustrations. Ellen has spent most of her adult years working in corporate America and has been extremely vigilant in balancing her work life and her health life. Ellen is proud to be the Vice President of the inaugural Board of Directors for Acromegaly Community.

The following article was previously published in the Daily Record *and is printed here with permission from the author, Lindy Korn, Esq.*

Genetic Bias in Workplace Made Illegal

On May 21st, 2008 President Bush signed into law (H.R. 493), The Genetic Information Nondiscrimination Act (GINA) ,which prohibits employers from discharging, refusing to hire, or otherwise discriminating against employees on the basis of genetic information. It applies to employment agencies and labor unions as well. The law also amends ERISA to preclude group health plans and health insurance issuers from discriminating against individuals based on genetic information, and it prohibits insurers from requiring genetic tests.

The act specifically exempts employers who obtain such information under the FMLA processes. However, employers have expressed concern about the prospect of liability when the employer did not solicit or intend to obtain such data. For example, what if an employee requests a leave (other than under FMLA), to care for her mother who has breast cancer or though conversations with a manager about an employee's parents disease? These issues will probably be the cause of new litigation.

The ADA is another area for concern. While accommodating an employee's disability via an interactive process, the employer may acquire genetic information without any intent to do so. GINA does provide that an employer's "inadvertent" acquisition of genetic information would not expose the employer to potential liability. The scope of the protection seems at this juncture to be vague, since "inadvertent" depends on the context. For example, if a manager visits a sick employee in the hospital and learns that the employee's malady has a genetic basis, would that information be obtained "inadvertently"?

GINA does provide for a private right of action, with jury trial and compensatory and punitive damages patterned after Title VII of the 1964 Civil Rights Act. The need for GINA arose in response to employee's fear of participating in clinical trials or to undergo genetic tests because of the fear that employers or health insurers would discriminate against them.

GINA's employment title takes effect 18 months after enactment and the act requires the EEOC to issue final regulations within a year of enactment. Hopefully the regulations will assist with state laws banning genetic data discrimination and their interplay with GINA.

GINA represents a win for privacy advocates and opens a Pandora's Box for employers!

Three Steps to Empowerment to Move Your Health Control to ForwardFast.

Mark Stinson

As I write this, I have in mind all who are facing a tough medical challenge. It may be someone who is newly diagnosed and looking for information. It may be those considering their treatment options and seeking some emotional support from others who have been there. Or it may be family members (or even employers) trying to offer encouragement and assistance in a meaningful way.

The starting point of improved health has always been the same: it begins with a sense of empowerment. There is nothing more important and nothing that improves the odds more than casting off negative limitations.

"The secret of health
for both mind and body
is not to mourn for the past,
nor to worry about the future,
but to live the present moment
wisely and earnestly."

- Buddha

Living in the moment is something all of us work on. But in this chapter, I'd like to focus on the "wisely and earnestly" part of that quote. What can you do to feel more empowered? How can you become wiser in your knowledge? More earnest in your actions? They are within your control.

Throughout my career as a medical communications professional, I have been driven to accelerate the use of new medical treatments to improve the quality of life of people who are suffering. And people with disease, with pain, or with disability can't wait. So my wake up call every day is to move with urgency to learn fast, track fast, think fast, respond fast, and create fast. *ForwardFast.*

For me, that is my focus of living in the now. And that's why right now I want to leverage all my experience and skills in education, communications, and persuasion—all to help people like you feel more empowered.

With the passion I have for what I'm doing—this passion for advancing medicine—I actually gain energy from being on the move.

A lot of people might tell you to slow down. Or they might say you're rushing things. Or that "we need more time." And certainly, there will be times when we can enjoy rewinding, going back to reminisce and relive an experience. But then, it's time to restart. If you want to take more control of your health, you must work extra hard to be very creatively prepared and focused to related to the science, the medical research, the physicians, the nurses, the clinics, the fellow patients, and the other people needed for the best outcomes.

And the journey can be measured not simply by speed, but by outcome. I've seen the value this empowered approach can create in people's lives. The fact that it can touch so many people, so fast, gives new meaning to medical advancement.

So that's why I can't sit still.

I'm living at the speed of hope.

I've had the opportunity to work with a company changing kidney dialysis and another with a revolutionary device to transport kidneys for transplant. In both cases, we were working to completely change the current practice of medicine and replace older technologies. In fact, the kidney transport device was featured in *Business Week* magazine as one of the "Ten Devices Changing Medicine." With the promise of simpler routines, improved quality of life, and even better survival, we can be motivated to live in *ForwardFast*... now.

One foundation we helped brand is delivering hope to those with arthritis, and another is improving the way hospital labs identify diseases faster. Both have strong clinical evidence of a "better way" to help people who would otherwise suffer needlessly. So, we work to communicate the news in *ForwardFast* ... now.

One of my clients is working on cellular therapy for cardiovascular diseases, while another is bringing the first approved treatment for a rare disease caused by a genetic disorder in the blood. Both have been years in development, so every day we help speed up the development processes—and get these life-changing treatments on the market—can make a dramatic difference for patients and their families. So, we live in *ForwardFast* ... now.

One of our diagnostic company clients wants to get the word out that they have a better way to diagnose ovarian cancer. And with another company, we need to accelerate the awareness of a treatment algorithm for sleep apnea, an often-underappreciated cause of cardiovascular disease. So, living in the now means working in *ForwardFast*.

In the world, you can look around and see the people who take this empowered approach. They are the ones who are

- making significant changes about how they view their health,
- choosing their attitudes with purpose,
- taking charge of their medical and lifestyle choices,
- seeking out the right healthcare professionals to create teams that support their personal outcomes, and
- taking action to make things happen.

So, now take a look at your own world. Let's consider what you can learn from others' outcomes. And what you have the power to do.

Let's reduce it down to 3 A's:

- ASK
- ATTITUDE
- ACTION

- ASK

Ask and you shall receive. How many times have you heard that? But how many times have you used this fundamental truth in your daily life recently?

My friend and mentor, Jack Canfield,* calls this the "Aladdin Principle."

I can't tell you how often smart people – confronting difficult situations and facing tough medical challenges – falter because they simply stop practicing the art of asking. In other words, we must know when and how to ask the right questions to gather the right information, seek useful referrals, generate new treatment ideas, and expand the options available.

If the simple act of asking is so critical, then why don't more people do it?

Because for some reason, people falsely think asking implies weakness. Or perhaps because it might signal distrust of the medical professionals we rely on. It's easy to come up with all sorts of excuses to avoid asking questions that can return unexpected or critical answers. Yet the world responds to those who ask. If you are not moving closer to what you want, you probably aren't doing enough asking.

Here are seven asking strategies (I learned by asking Jack Canfield) that you can implement in your life to potentially boost your confidence:

1. Ask for Information

You can never have too much information. To gain potentially life-changing insights, you first need to have an understanding about the current challenges, what might be accomplished, and the plan to treat it. Only then can you proceed with empowerment. Ask questions starting with the words who, why, what, where, when and how to obtain the information you need. When you truly understand the situation, you can better appreciate a solution.

2. Ask for Time

You know how pressed for time you feel when talking with a doctor. And the doctor is under pressure to see more patients. It's the nature of the system (if you can still call healthcare today a "system"). Always ask the questions you want. Don't waffle or talk around it – or worse, wait for your doctor to leave. No doubt you have heard of many good ways to ask the question, "Could I get more time to talk to you or someone about this?" The point is, ask.

3. Ask for Expert Introductions

These can be difficult to ask for if you don't feel you "deserve" to talk to more experienced professionals. But asking to be introduced to highly respected experts is a powerful tool. It can solidify the quality of your care plan and leverage your connections to even more people with integrity, trustworthiness, and the ability to get you what you need. When is the best time to ask? Right after you have had an excellent discussion with your doctor. Simply ask if your physician would be willing to give you an introduction to a renowned expert in the field – someone from whom you could learn more.

4. Ask for Top-Quality Referrals

Just about everyone knows the importance of referrals. If you need the support of other specialists or allied health professionals or exercise physiologist or nutritionist, start by asking. In fact, there's a popular way of asking, "If it were your family member, who would you go to?" It's the easiest, most direct way of ensuring you get the best possible recommendation. And frankly, if all the recommendations are within the same hospital or health system network, you can keep asking, "Are they the best in this hospital or the best overall?"

5. Ask for More Time

Before I talked about asking for longer time during your appointment. Now, you still need more time – time to do your homework, time to talk to experts, time to reflect and think. This doesn't mean delaying decisions just to put them off, but don't be rushed into a treatment direction.

6. Ask for Feedback

This is an important component of asking that is often overlooked. How do you really know if your compliance to therapy is meeting expectations? Ask your doctor, "How am I doing? What can I do to improve my end of the bargain? How can I better fulfill my commitment? Please share with me what you like or don't like about what I'm doing." By setting up this kind of honest conversation, you're opening up a way to ask good questions and tough questions. It's a powerful way to fine-tune your health regimen.

7. Ask to Renegotiate

Even in global diplomatic stalemates, rarely is the negotiating room ever locked for good. The same should be true of your treatment plan. It may involve negotiation and often re-negotiation, which is simply another form of asking that could save a lot of time, frustration, and perhaps, money. As long as your doctor knows you're negotiating in a positive spirit, you can enjoy a lot of flexibility. Nothing is ever cast in stone. It's only in stone if you don't speak up!

- ATTITUDE

The thing you have the most control of is, first and foremost, your attitude. Many of the other stories shared in this book can give you a sense of motivation. So, maybe I can help add to that a sense of empowerment. There may not be some secret that can guarantee you results, however big or small. But if you ever find yourself hitting brick walls and coming up short, come back to these attitude tips:

- Clarity: Be precise. Think clearly about your request. Take time to prepare. Use a note pad to pick words that have the greatest impact. Words are powerful, so choose them carefully. No one likes getting a vague or fuzzy question. For example, if you throw out the "How am I doing?" question without specifics, it may take time for the other person to understand what you're talking about. Instead, try, "How is my attitude with my family? Do you see room for improvement? How?"

- Confidence: People who exhibit confidence get more than those who are hesitant and uncertain. When you've figured out what you want, do it with certainty, boldness and confidence. Practice in the mirror if you have to. Be prepared to hear the unexpected or the unwanted. Try to have an open mind and heart (it's okay to feel intimidated by the experience, but don't show it). Don't get defensive if you hear something you don't like or that makes you uncomfortable. It's good to get a little uneasy once in a while upon the observations or insights of others. They will inspire you to stop, reflect, and take steps to make a shift for the better.

- Consistency: Empowered patients know that they can't quit if they try once and don't get a good response. Keep working at it until you find the answers, and try different ways if one doesn't seem to be working. In any treatment, there are usually four or five "no's" before you get a "yes."

- Creativity: In this age of health, science, and technology innovation, the answer you need might go undiscovered. If you want someone's attention – if you want some more information – don't simply stop with the ordinary way. Use your creativity to dream up another approach. Here's one way to engage the insights of a valued expert or even a peer: "I highly value your opinion and honest perspective and would love to know what you think I could be doing differently on a daily basis that would make my life easier and make a difference in my condition."

- Sincerity: When you really need help, people will respond. Sincerity means dropping the image facade and showing a willingness to be vulnerable. Tell it the way it is, lumps and all. Don't worry if your presentation isn't perfect; ask from your heart. Keep it simple and people will open up to you. I trust you'll be surprised and delighted at what you discover about yourself in this process.

- ACTION

When you have more knowledge from asking, and you've improved your attitude, now can feel more empowered to take action. Talking with your doctor and following the prescribed plan are two of the most important elements of taking control of your health.

Here are some actions you can take to achieve better results from both of those:

Prepare your list of questions and concerns.

Before your appointment, write a list of what you want to ask. In the waiting room, review your list and organize your thoughts. Even share the list with your doctor or nurse.

Describe your symptoms.

Keep a notebook or diary to help you remember what happens between visits. When the problems started, and how they make you feel. If you know, write down what triggers them. And, on the other hand, what you have done to feel better.

Make a list of medications.

This should include all prescription drugs, along with over-the-counter medicines. Also, remember any vitamins, herbal products, and supplements. Everything matters and they can work together or they might be counter-productive.

Monitor your diet and lifestyle.

Daily eating habits and food selections can play important roles in overall health. Likewise, physical activity is a big contributor to your wellness. Consult your doctor about smoking, alcohol intake, or drug use. Finally, be frank about your sexual history and current activities, as these are another indicator of your well-being.

Learn about tests.

Be prepared to receive specific instructions on any medical tests and what you need to do to get ready for them. Be sure to understand any risks or side effects of the test. And be clear about how and when you can get the test results. This will all give you a greater sense of assurance, instead of worry.

Discuss treatments and options.

Of course, this starts from the time of initial therapy. But it continues through changes in dosing or frequency, or even switching medications. Consider newly available products and weigh your choices carefully.

Align with the plan.

I had a physician share with me recently his views on different terms used to describe patients' behaviors on medical recommendations: "adherence," "compliance," and "concordance." Eventually, the issue of compliance is really one of implementation and execution. For what it's worth, he says, "alignment" is a better premise. We are not striving to persuade, coerce, or trick patients into doing what their doctors prescribe. But rather to align clinicians, patients, payers, and anyone else involved in healthcare so that everyone is working in concert. An easy example of *alignment*'s advantages is the case in which a patient does not adhere to the prescribed treatment plan, but does communicate that decision and her reasons to the clinicians. That is not "compliance" (at least by a strict definition), but it seems different from and more preferable to the case in which the patient not only does not follow the treatment plan, but also misleads the clinician into thinking he is doing so. Assuming the patient was not just perversely turning down all options, he or she and the clinicians could be in "alignment" although the patient is not in "compliance."

In conclusion, you and your physician make up a team – and you play a powerful role on that team. As one physician tells her patients, "I'm going to try to be the best doctor I can and prescribe the right things and teach you about the disease. And you're going to try to learn about your body and how you're feeling and come in and be honest and tell me what you're experiencing."

I've shared with you steps to take control of your health by talking with your doctor and following the prescribed plan. I suggested adding to your sense of empowerment – and motivation – with specific ways to improve your attitude. And I proposed that asking the right questions would help you gather the right information, seek useful referrals, generate new treatment ideas, and expand the options available. All these, in my experience, are making significant changes about how people view their health.

And I hope you'll consider applying them to move your health forward…fast.

Mark Stinson is a medical writer and strategic facilitator. His consultancy, STINSON Brand Innovation, serves clients in all sectors of health, science, and technology. Mark conducts healthcare professional workshops, new product development initiatives, communication tool presentations, and teleseminars. Mark's career in medical communications spans some 30 years. Mark received a communications degree from Louisiana State University. He and his wife Jenny divide their time between homes in the Chicago neighborhood of Roscoe Village and in Boise, Idaho. *ForwardFast* is a registered trademark of Stinson Brand Innovation, Inc.

* Jack Canfield, America's #1 Success Coach, is founder of the billion-dollar book brand *Chicken Soup for the Soul* and a leading authority on Peak Performance and Life Success. His bestselling book, *The Success Principles: How to Get from Where You Are to Where You Want to Be* contains dozens of the most powerful secrets to success used by top achievers from all walks of life.

Psychological Aspects of Acromegaly

Valerie Golden, PhD, LP

Introduction

Patients with Acromegaly often ask whether they will ever again live a normal life. The answer is yes, absolutely, but perhaps a "new normal." It takes time to integrate physical changes, face emotional challenges, adapt to change, and create a satisfying life; it also requires an active approach to problem solving.

As Acromegaly affects patients physically, it also affects patients psychologically, specifically in terms of emotions, confidence, self-image, and overall sense of well-being. Too often the powerful psychological impact is not fully acknowledged.

Achieving a normal life means accepting some aspects, finding ways to feel more in control, making educated and informed decisions, adapting to both physical and emotional changes, redefining priorities, and actively processing what may have been lost in order to make room for new gains. It also means staying connected to what makes your particular life enjoyable and meaningful to you. It may sound formidable, but yes, absolutely, patients can create not only normal lives, but also in many instances lives of even greater meaning and purpose.

Emotions and Acromegaly

Within the spectrum of what is normal, individuals vary greatly in their emotional temperaments, stress tolerance, and preferred coping styles. For patients with Acromegaly, the most frequent emotional hurdles involve anger, depression, and irritability.

Remember that diagnosis and treatment themselves are anxiety provoking events, giving rise to fears about pain, finances, job stability, long term job performance, body changes, and relationship issues, in addition to apprehension about potential neurosurgery. And that's just for patients! Family members and others close to the patient also experience fear and anxiety with the diagnosis.

Some respond to Acromegaly with social isolation/withdrawal, loss of libido, lowered self-esteem, regressive behaviors, and displacement. Regression may manifest as becoming more needy and childlike, perhaps to enlist others' help or support. Displacement involves taking out anger and frustration on others, often those closest to the patient because they are "safe," rather than more directly on the source/target of frustration. Both regression and displacement may occur because the angry feelings are hard to express in words or because the patient feels unable to direct the anger directly at the more appropriate real target, as in the case of illness, death, natural disaster, or the like.

These reactions may be difficult to tolerate in oneself, one's partner, or one's grown child. Try to understand these behaviors as your (or the patient's) best efforts to cope with fears and anxieties, at least for right now.

Mourning for Loss

Diagnosis is life changing and an illness is a loss. There may be a loss of the pre-diagnosis self, loss of self-mastery, loss of former self-image, loss of one's "old" face/hands/feet, loss of being perfectly healthy, and maybe even loss of feeling invincible (e.g., "it won't happen to me"). Grief is a natural response to loss.

Remember, however, that everyone grieves in his or her own way. There is no neat, linear, one-size-fits-all, sequential path. Some skip whole stages altogether, healing without ever experiencing a particular phase. For most, there is a back-and-forth movement among stages, with considerable overlap, as they move through the process.

That said, typical responses to grief and loss involve the following stages:

<u>Resignation:</u> This differs from acceptance. The individual often feels helpless and unable to take control.

<u>Denial:</u> Shock, disbelief, numbness. "This can't be happening to me."

<u>Anger:</u> "Why me? What/Who can I blame?"

<u>Bargaining</u>: "Please make it not so and I'll do anything in return."

<u>Depression:</u> "I'm too sad to do anything." May include resignation.

<u>Acceptance and Adaptation</u>: "I can come to terms with this. I will regain control in these helpful, adaptive ways."

It is important to distinguish between normal grief and depression (which requires professional treatment). Grief comes in waves similar to a roller coaster ride; depression feels constant. Feelings of despair, emptiness, hopelessness, and worthlessness are hallmarks of depression. If there are thoughts of suicide and an inability to function at work, home, or school, it may be depression rather than normal grief over loss. Drug or alcohol abuse, or self neglect (e.g., poor personal hygiene) may point to depression rather than normal grief. If you suspect depression, remember that it is treatable and seek the help of a mental health professional.

How to Cope

While lots of factors influence the ability to cope with Acromegaly (e.g., personality traits, family support, education, social status), the biggest factor is whether the individual has an avoidant/passive or an active coping style.

An active coping style involves solving problems for yourself, (i.e., taking charge, planning, anticipating potential challenges and working around them). Competence and control are the greatest antidotes to anxiety.

For example, identifying a potentially embarrassing social situation or remark, and planning what to say or how to handle it should it arise can restore a sense of confidence, effectiveness, and agency. Competence and control diminish anxiety because in most instances anxiety is really a worry that "I won't be able to handle it if *x* happens." By actively developing solutions in advance, you can face otherwise tough situations with increased comfort, not to mention skill.

Illness often requires you to give up control of certain parts of your life. It's normal to feel angry about losing any self-mastery; however, it is both possible and essential to find new ways of regaining control.

Highly Effective Strategies Include:
1.Active Problem Solving:
Again, competence and control. Key aspects are

a. Knowledge and Information: learn about Acromegaly so you can be an effective participant in your own care and make decisions about available options.
b. Planning: anticipate hurdles and ways to minimize problems. Know your triggers and plan around them.
c. Realistic goals: take small steps in the right direction and you will get there.
d. Flexibility. If your first try doesn't work, reassess and adjust.
e. Humor: maintain your sense of humor.
f. Redefining your self-worth as needed. For example, if appearance was too far up on your list of defining factors, identify other aspects to like about yourself. Remember, at your funeral, no one will be talking about your ring size or tooth gaps; rather they will talk about how you lived your life and what you meant to others.

Active problem solving means facing issues; avoidance only fosters more fear and anxiety.

2. Cognitive Restructuring:
Restructure the way you talk to yourself. For example, reassure yourself that you can do something to generate solutions.

a. Avoid catastrophic thinking. Rather, think realistically (e.g., instead of "the world will end," tell yourself "in the worst case scenario, I could do this . . .").
b. Avoid all-or-nothing thinking (e.g., "If I don't do everything perfectly, I am a total failure" can be made significantly more helpful as "I have the following strengths I can bring to bear").

3. Self Care:

a. Face feelings.
b. Reduce stress.
c. Maintain proper diet and exercise.
d. Get adequate rest and relaxation.
e. Manage your time and energy.
f. Communicate your needs directly. People are not good mind readers.
g. Identify sources of strength (e.g., people, activities, solitude, nature, etc.) in which you take pride.
h. Distract yourself when stress mounts.
i. Stay connected to what's enjoyable and meaningful to you.
j. To the greatest extent possible, design the life you want to live (find meaning and purpose in what interests you and makes you feel useful, worthwhile, happy, and connected to others).

Anger Management

Many people with Acromegaly struggle with anger and its effects, frequently requesting help targeted specifically to anger management. While there is overlap between anger management strategies and other coping strategies discussed above (e.g., problem solving, competence and control are helpful in anger management, too), the following strategies target anger management in particular:

1. Become a Better Communicator.

Slowing down instead of spouting off the moment you feel upset can be hugely important. Anger makes us all jump to conclusions that are often exaggerated and unrealistic. Interjecting some time gives you greater control and assures that you say what you really want to say rather than something you may later regret. Instead of saying the first thing that comes into your head in the heat of the moment, tell yourself to "strike when the iron is cool," giving yourself the chance to reflect on your behavior and its potential consequences. Remember, you can always say it later, in 5 minutes, an hour, a day, a week . . . but you can't always take it back. The increased self-control will not only improve relationships, but also bolster your self-esteem.

Improve your communication skills further by learning to express yourself in more realistic and accurate terms. When anger strikes, we tend to think in absolutes. Avoid terms like "never" and "always." It's not true that your spouse "always" ignores you, or "never" understands you. Such words not only justify your anger to yourself and even fuel more anger, they also alienate others, putting them on the defensive rather than enlisting their help in problem solving.

Learn to listen to what others are saying and focus on the underlying feelings they are expressing. Often if you can rephrase your spouse's demands for more of your time and attention as a desire for closeness, you can dissipate the anger. By contrast, labeling him or her as your jailer will fuel more anger and misunderstanding. By communicating your attempts to hear what is being said and understand the other's perspective, you forestall defensiveness and impasses.

2. Relax.

Simple relaxation strategies such as deep breathing (from the diaphragm) and visualizing relaxing scenes/experiences can calm you down when anger strikes. Yoga and meditation also help.

Perhaps most important of all, make time for whatever replenishes your energy and vitality, be it yoga, meditation, solitude, guided imagery, music, travel, social events, reading, or hobbies.

Remember that Acromegaly can cause sleep apnea, too, which can lead to anger, irritability, and serious health risks if untreated. Get adequate rest and relaxation, and if you suspect sleep apnea, get evaluated and treated.

3. Reframe Angry Thoughts and Self-Talk.

Anger tends to elicit dramatic and exaggerated emotions and self talk. Instead of "Oh, this is just horrible and all is lost" try "this is frustrating and inconvenient but not a tragedy, certainly not the end of the world, and I'm going to slow myself down to think."

4. Use Logic to Defeat Anger.

Logic defeats anger, because anger quickly becomes irrational. Tell yourself the world is not conspiring to make you miserable; instead, you've hit a normal bump along the way. Instead of demanding your due (e.g., fairness, appreciation, agreement, flexibility) from others, translate your demands into desires rather than entitlements. Restructure your cognitions to become aware of demands, reframing "I absolutely must have" into "I would like." Others will take notice and in turn respond more positively to you. Even if they can't give you what you want, the interaction will be more harmonious. Sometimes disappointment and hurt are inevitable, but they are never helped by irrational anger.

5. Continue to Problem Solve for Self-Respect.

When facing the real and inevitable problems of daily life, especially ones you can't solve, you may also feel anger and frustration—as a natural, healthy, rational response. Continue to problem solve, to aim for solutions, and find self-respect in giving it your best efforts, in trying to face matters head on, even if the problem isn't one you can solve.

6. Defuse with Humor.

Use humor to defuse the situation and restore equilibrium, to remind yourself that what angers you is not the end of the world. Be careful, however, that you don't use humor to mask underlying sarcasm or hostility.

7. Change Your Environment.

Change what you can in your environment to facilitate your anger management goals. For example, if you know that certain times of day are stressful, build in some stress relief or relaxation then. Certainly avoid discussions of volatile emotional conflicts at times you know you are emotionally spread thin. If you know certain people, places, or situations upset you, ask yourself if it's an involvement you might realistically avoid; seek alternatives that help you stay calm; distract yourself from stress and anger when you can.

Conclusion

Taking an active approach to problem solving and reframing one's internal dialogue are highly effective ways of dealing with the emotional aspects of Acromegaly, as well as other life stressors.

In doing so, people often find strengths they never knew they had. For example, refocusing on what's really important in relationships can mean becoming a better friend, partner, parent, employee, neighbor, or family member. Dealing with illness can lead us to reassess priorities, which in turn can move us toward living life to the fullest, with greater focus on what's truly important to us . . . a life that's ultimately more successful in our own terms.

Valerie Golden, Ph.D., is a Clinical Psychologist in Minneapolis, MN. She received her undergraduate degree from Stanford University and her Ph.D. in clinical psychology from Columbia University where, following graduation, she served on the adjunct faculty of Columbia University's Program in Clinical Psychology as well as the mental health staff at Columbia University. She currently serves on the Executive Steering Committee of the Affiliate Council of the American Psychoanalytic Association and is a member of the MN

Psychological Association, the American Psychological Association, the American Psychoanalytic Association, and the Minnesota Psychoanalytic Society & Institute. She has lectured nationwide at medical conferences on pituitary disease, including at Harvard University, Stanford University, and the University of VA. She has also contributed to popular press articles such as *Psychology Today.*

Epilogue

On behalf of all of our wonderful authors, I would like to personally thank you for taking this trip with us through our many adventures and misadventures in the medical universe, family management, and *life*. While not all of the stories were happy stories, we all continue to battle every day to make sure we come out on top. Life journeys are rarely always easy or pleasant, but it is from those greatest hardships that we have the greatest opportunity to grow. When personal struggles befall you, make sure you take the information as a life lesson and work to overcome residual pain; it is from this combination that the most growth comes. I hope our stories of hardship, occasional failure, and eventual victory inspire you to do the same with your own life and your own struggles.

Editing this book has been the single greatest opportunity of my life. I am so honored to have gotten the chance to work with these great authors. Please understand that we have all poured our hearts onto the pages that fill this book, and my working with all of them to help unite our voices into one resounding voice of strength has been overwhelming.

I know that I learned a lot as I wrote my own chapter, and judging by the feedback from the other writers, they felt the same about their chapters as well. As I read their chapters to put the book together, I found myself learning about myself from other people's experiences.

There is a common belief that all patients dealing with Acromegaly have totally different symptoms. But I am sure that as you read, the thread became clear to you; as it did to me. This disease is a magnifier. That is why the symptoms always seem so unique. We are not talking about a cold or flu with achiness and sniffles. We are talking about a disease that just magnifies whatever is going on in your life. If you are already an emotional person, this disease will make you far more emotional. If you are someone prone to anger or short-temperedness, this is going to become far more apparent. Our job, as patients, is to try to work the hardest to manage our emotions when we feel most crummy. Conversely, we do ask that our loved ones be understanding on the odd time that we are not successful in achieving this goal. Please love us, even if it is in spite of ourselves, sometimes. We are doing our best to control our emotions.

If you are a patient dealing with the effects of Acromegaly, I hope that this book brought you strength to keep going. Remember, some days are better than others, but no matter what, you are NOT alone! There is a huge universe filled with wonderful people who would love to help you along your path.

If you are a loved one of someone managing Acromegaly, I hope that you were able to understand a little bit more of how we live and manage our lives. This is not always the easiest disease to manage, and sometimes we may struggle on our journey, but we are trying to make the best of it all.

Finally, I know that as patients, sometimes we do not always remember to express our appreciation to our loved ones enough. I would like to take this last opportunity to thank all the wonderful people who we deal with on a regular basis … who deal with our good days and our bad ones... who love us when we feel most unlovable … who are there in the hospital with us holding our hands… who help us with our medical procedures. Your love and generosity is truly valued and appreciated. Our lives are richer because you are in them. We love you and we thank you for everything you are to us.

For More Information

Because information on the Internet can be somewhat transitional, and links change and move all the time, if you would like to learn more about Acromegaly, or how to support people with rare diseases, please go to AcromegalyCommunity.com.

Thank you for reading our stories. We hope that you found them informative and interesting.